WORLD BANK TECHNICAL PAPER NO. 326

Africa Technical Department Series

The Condition of Young Children in Sub-Saharan Africa

The Convergence of Health, Nutrition, and Early Education

Nat J. Colletta
Jayshree Balachander
Xioyan Liang

The World Bank
Washington, D.C.

Technical Papers are published to communicate the results of the Bank's work to the development community with the least possible delay. The typescript of this paper therefore has not been prepared in accordance with the procedures appropriate to formal printed texts, and the World Bank accepts no responsibility for errors. Some sources cited in this paper may be informal documents that are not readily available.

The complete backlist of publications from the World Bank is shown in the annual Index of Publications, which contains an alphabetical title list (with full ordering information) and indexes of subjects, authors, and countries and regions. The latest edition is available free of charge from the Distribution Unit, Office of the Publisher, The World Bank, 1818 H Street, N.W., Washington, D.C. 20433, U.S.A., or from Publications, The World Bank, 66, avenue d'Iéna, 75116 Paris, France.

ISSN: 0253-7494

The cover panel was designed by Jennifer Sterling. The photos are by Curt Carnemark, The World Bank; the National Center for Early Childhood Education, Kenya; and Nat J. Colletta.

In the World Bank's Africa Technical Department, Nat J. Colletta is principal education and social policy specialist and Jayshree Balachander is senior nutrition specialist. Xiaoyan Liang is a child development specialist and research assistant in the World Bank's Human Development Department.

Library of Congress Cataloging-in-Publication Data

Colletta, Nat J.
    The condition of young children in Sub-Saharan Africa : the
convergence of health, nutrition, and early education / Nat J.
Colletta, Jayshree Balachander, and Xiaoyan Liang.
       p.   cm. — (World Bank technical paper, ISSN 0253-7494 ; no.
326) (World Bank technical paper. Africa Technical Department
series)
  Includes bibliographical references (p.).
  ISBN 0-8213-3677-0
  1. Children—Africa, Sub-Saharan. 2. Poor children—Africa, Sub-
Saharan. 3. Children—Health and hygiene—Africa, Sub-Saharan.
4. Children—Services for —Africa, Sub-Saharan. 5. Fundamental
education—Africa, Sub-Saharan. 6. Child development—Africa, Sub-
Saharan. 7. Africa, Sub-Saharan—Social conditions—1960–
I. Balachander, Jayshree, 1957– . II. Liang, Xiaoyan.
III. Title. IV. Series. V. Series: World Bank technical paper.
Africa Technical Department series.
HQ792.A4C57 1996
305.23'0967—dc20
                                     96-25649
                                      CIP

AFRICA TECHNICAL DEPARTMENT PAPERS

Technical Paper Series

Discussion Paper Series

CONTENTS

BOXES

FOREWORD

Of the world's two billion young children below the age of 14, about 12 percent are from the 47 countries that comprise the Sub-Saharan region of Africa (SSA). However, of the 40,000 children that die everyday in the world, nearly 30 percent are African. The burden of debt, economic mismanagement and recession, civil strife, pandemic disease, and natural calamities have combined to weaken the resource base for investing in Africa's children. How does the condition of African children fare compared with children in other parts of the world? What is happening to them in terms of survival, health, nutrition, and early childhood development? What can be done to improve their condition?

The Africa Region has been working closely with UNICEF, the Aga Khan Foundation, the Van Leer Foundation, Save the Children, USAID, the Consultative Group on Early Childhood Education, and other partners to promote the development of the young African child through comprehensive sector approaches in health, nutrition, and education.

This study draws attention to the plight of the African child, particularly the much-neglected period between birth/infancy and primary school entry (or early childhood), by first describing the broad socioeconomic and demographic trends over the last decade on the African continent, then by examining the current condition of the young African child as shaped by these trends. Moving beyond the overview, it proceeds to summarize current thinking on how early childhood development (ECD) programs might contribute to breaking the intergenerational cycle of poverty on the African continent. It emphasizes that timely intervention is crucial in this regard.

The Africa ECD Initiative entails a three-pronged strategy of: *(a)* knowledge generation and dissemination; *(b)* prototype program development; and *(c)* capacity building. This study is the first in a series of products from the Africa Regional Early Childhood Development Initiative. A second study on the overall ECD policy and programmatic effort (government and non-governmental) in Africa is currently under preparation. Country case studies are also under way in South Africa, Kenya, and Mauritius, where a rich array of alternative delivery systems, financing schemes, and quality enhancement programs are being tested. In the capacity building arena, an African ECD Network comprising practitioners and policymakers representing some 21 countries has been formed and is seeking formal recognition as a Working Group within the Association for the Development of African Education (DAE).

Kevin Cleaver
Director
Technical Department
Africa Region

ABSTRACT

In Sub-Saharan Africa, a number of adverse conditions have placed children at high risk, including persistent and worsening poverty, an alarming pace of economic change, rapid population growth, increasing urbanization, a changing family structure, and growing numbers of orphaned refugees and displaced women and children from internal civil strife, among other things. For many children, primary school interventions are too late to prevent irreversible disability or to allow for the development of full adult capacity. The focus on a viable social policy for children under five is an urgent necessity.

This first product of the Africa Region's Initiative on Early Childhood Development (ECD) describes the condition of young children in Africa, calls attention to their plight, and begins to explore strategies to address their condition. The ECD initiative focuses on the neglected but critical developmental age group between birth and school enrollment and views child development not as an extension of traditional schooling downward, but as the 'holistic' development of the child. It envisages the integration of physical, cognitive, and socioemotional development as a necessary foundation for full growth and maturation and entails a three-pronged strategy: to generate and disseminate knowledge, develop prototype programs, and build institutional capacity, focusing especially on expanding the traditional role of the female child beyond that of caregiver. This report on the status of the African child will be followed by an assessment of the policy, programmatic, and financial efforts of African governments, NGOs, private citizens, and donors to address the needs of the young African child, as well as in-depth country studies and innovative prototype ECD programs.

ACKNOWLEDGMENTS

The authors wish to acknowledge the guidance provided by an advisory group consisting of the following persons: Samuel Lieberman, Principal Human Resource Economist, EA2PH, Mary E. Young, Senior PHN Specialist, HDD, and Margaret Grieco, Social Scientist, Gender Team, AFTHR. External reviews were provided by Ash Hartwell, Education Specialist, USAID, Washington; Linda Biersteker, Child Research Specialist, Early Learning Resource Unit, South Africa; and Fred Woods, Director, Early Beginnings Program, Save the Children, USA. The Managing Division Chief is Ishrat Husain, AFTHR, and the Department Director is Kevin Cleaver, AFTDR. P.C. Mohan provided editorial assistance and Elizabeth Acul typed the final document.

ABBREVIATIONS

ALC	Active Learning Capacity
ECD	Early Childhood Development
DHS	Demographic and Health Surveys
DPT	Diphtheria, Pertussis, and Tetanus
HDI	Human Development Index
IFPRI	International Food Policy Research Institute
IMR	Infant Mortality Rate
GER	Gross Enrollment Ratio
NGO	Non-Governmental Organization
OECD	Organization for Economic Cooperation and Development
ORT	Oral Rehydration Therapy
SSA	Sub-Saharan Africa
TB	Tuberculosis
UNDP	United Nations Development Program
UNESCO	United Nations Educational, Scientific and Cultural Organization
UNICEF	United Nations Children's Fund
UNHCR	United Nations High Commissioner for Refugees
WIC	Supplemental Nutrition Program for Women, Infants, and Children

EXECUTIVE SUMMARY

For many children in Sub-Saharan Africa, primary school interventions are already too late to prevent irreversible disability or to allow for the development of full adult capacity. Infant mortality in the region is one-and-a-half times that of the world average of 60 per thousand and over three times that of the European and Central Asian rate of 30 per thousand. About 30 percent of children under 5 suffer from chronic malnutrition. Under 5 mortality is two times higher than the world average of 173 per thousand and four times that of the European and Central Asian rate of 75 per thousand. Only 63 percent of the region's children have been immunized against tuberculosis and less than 50 percent against DPT, polio and measles.

Beyond the age of 5 an African child's chances of entering a primary school are less than 50 percent, of completing primary school, less than 35 percent, of finishing secondary school, less than 12 percent and of entering university under 2 percent. Many of the same conditions of poverty that previously placed the under-5 at risk of death later leave them at risk of poor health, malnutrition and impaired mental, social and emotional development. In the age of globalization and increasing competition, these are alarming statistics.

Persistent poverty frames the plight of the African child. In the last decade while much of the world moved forward to improve the basic human condition, the degree of poverty in Africa actually worsened. The number of African families who were unable to meet their basic needs doubled in that period as average incomes fell by a third. In the same period, population grew by more than 40 percent, the fastest growing rate in the world (an average annual rate of 3 percent or nearly two-and-one-half times the world average rate of 1.7 percent). Africa today has the youngest population of any region in the world. This demographic explosion has disproportionately increased the numbers of children seeking access to basic services and food security. While the OECD countries, given their rapidly aging structure, shift their attention to social security and gerontology, in the Africa region, the focus on a viable social policy for young children is an urgent necessity.

As of 1992, Africa's GNP of $530 was among the lowest of all regions of the world. Income distribution paints an even bleaker picture. In 1994, the average African government's expenditure on defense (about 9 percent) was more than twice that on health. Utilizing UNDP's Human Development Index (a composite of literacy level, life expectancy, and consumptive power), 41 of the 54 lowest human development countries are in Sub-Saharan Africa.

This picture is compounded by rapid urbanization and the emerging breakdown of traditional family support structures. Labor migration, deterioration of rural infrastructure, unemployment, civil strife, and rapid social change have all begun to take their toll on the African family. Of the nearly 5 million orphans and 20 million refugees in Africa, 80 percent are female. It is estimated that nearly one-third of African households are now being headed by single women. These same women are being forced to carry the burden of earning an income, managing a household and caring for children with decreasing assistance. The vicious cycle of poverty is reproduced when young girls drop out of school (or never enter) in order to help in the household, lose their childhoods by becoming pregnant in their adolescent years, and end up trapped in poverty.

In sum, the uneven pace of economic change in Sub-Saharan Africa, its rapid population growth rate and increasing urbanization, the changing family structure, and growing numbers of orphaned refugees and displaced women and children from internal civil strife, among other things, has placed the African family in increased conditions of adversity and the child in a state of high risk and in need of urgent attention.

This study is the first product in the Africa Region's Initiative on Early Childhood Development. Its purpose is to describe the condition of young children in Africa, call attention to their plight, and begin the exploration of strategies to address their condition. While past global initiatives have focused on promoting Child Survival (through age one) and Universal Primary Education for All (beginning at age 5), this new initiative is concerned with the neglected, but critical developmental age group between birth and school enrollment. It sees child development not as an extension of traditional schooling downward often referred to as early childhood education or pre-school, but rather as the 'holistic' development of the child. It envisages the integration of physical, cognitive, and socioemotional development as a necessary foundation for full growth and maturation.

The first 5 years are a crucial period in the development of a child. Brain development is almost wholly completed by age 2 and malnutrition peaks at around 24 months of age. This implies the need for early interventions of health, nutrition, cognitive stimulation and socialization programs as a synergistic force, *converging* to promote the child's total development. It does not necessarily mean a single program or 'silver bullet,' but rather the mutual reinforcement of multiple program interventions in an efficient and cost-effective manner.

While we know much about efforts to achieve such child-centered impact in the industrial world, we know very little beyond the condition of the child on the African continent. The Africa Regional ECD Initiative entails a three-pronged strategy of knowledge building and dissemination, prototype program development, and capacity-institution building. This paper on the status of the Africa Child will be followed by an assessment of the policy, programmatic and financial efforts of African governments, NGOs, private citizens, and donors to address the needs of the young African child. In-depth country studies focusing on specific program models in select countries will be undertaken to learn from and leverage the existing experience in Africa across the continent. In parallel with these activities, the Bank will support innovative prototype ECD programs and projects such as the one recently appraised on Integrated ECD Services for the young Kenyan child. The third prong will entail a dissemination, training and capacity building program for African policymakers and practitioners, as well as Bank staff, in the design and implementation of cost-effective developmental interventions for young African children.

This initiative is undertaken in a context where gender is beginning to emerge on the policy horizon as a central developmental concern. The girl child has become a specific issue on the African change agenda. The initiative will explore ways of expanding the opportunity of the female child from her traditional and often limited role as care-giver in poor households.

Integrated or converging early childhood development programs should be seen as essential for a healthy, prosperous, creative and competitive environment. They can have a positive impact on child quality, school efficiency, economic productivity and social equity. Africa's future lies in ensuring that its children grow up in an environment where they can meet their full potential.

1. SOCIOECONOMIC INDICATORS AND TRENDS AFFECTING CHILD SURVIVAL AND DEVELOPMENT

> *A child is born without barriers. Its needs are integrated, and it is we who choose to compartmentalize them into health, nutrition, or education. Yet the child itself cannot isolate its hunger for food from its hunger for affection or its hunger for knowledge.* (Alava in Myers 1992a).

Poverty

Africa is a continent in transition, just beginning to pull out of decades of spiraling decline. Its children are at risk from drought, famine and civil strife. In the last decade when much of the world took great strides forward, improving basic human conditions, in Africa the degree of poverty actually worsened. The number of families in Sub-Saharan Africa who are unable to meet their basic needs doubled in that period as average incomes fell by a third. In the same period, population grew by more than 40 percent, swelling the ranks of the poor. To illustrate, in Cameroon, while fewer than 1 percent of households in the Yaoundé area fell below the poverty line in 1983, more than 20 percent of households did so in 1993 (World Bank 1995b). As of 1992, the SSA's regional average Gross National Product (GNP) per capita of 530 dollars was among the lowest of all the world regions (World Bank 1994a).

Of the countries with available data, the percent of the urban population living below the absolute poverty level ranges from 7 percent in Mali to as much as 31 percent in Zambia, with an average of about 14 percent living in absolute poverty in 1991. The situation in rural areas is even worse. The proportion of the rural population living in absolute poverty averages 45 percent, ranging from 24 percent in Cameroon to 85 percent in Malawi.[1]

In some countries, while the percentage of population in poverty remained largely unchanged during the last decade, the depth of poverty actually increased. For instance, Kenya had about 47 percent of its population living under poverty in the last decade, but the shortfall of average income of the poor below the poverty line increased from 30 percent to 40 percent in 1992 (World Bank 1995b).

The poor have the least access to basic health, education and social services. Children from poor families are more likely to be sick and malnourished, and less likely to attend school than those from better-off families. During the critical formative years of rapid growth, such deprivation often has consequences that are long-lasting and often irreversible, affecting their ability to perform in school, and resulting often in failure in their adult lives. Furthermore, poverty is also intertwined with inadequate parenting skills for formal schooling or preparing

---

[1] World Bank 1995a. Absolute poverty is defined as the country-specific income level below which adequate standards of nutrition, shelter, and personal amenities cannot be assured (UNDP 1993 and World Bank data). See Annex 1 for a list of the countries comprising Sub-Saharan Africa.

children for new types of jobs. Low literacy levels reduce access to information and public resources.

Figure 1: Percentage of Population Living under Absolute Poverty

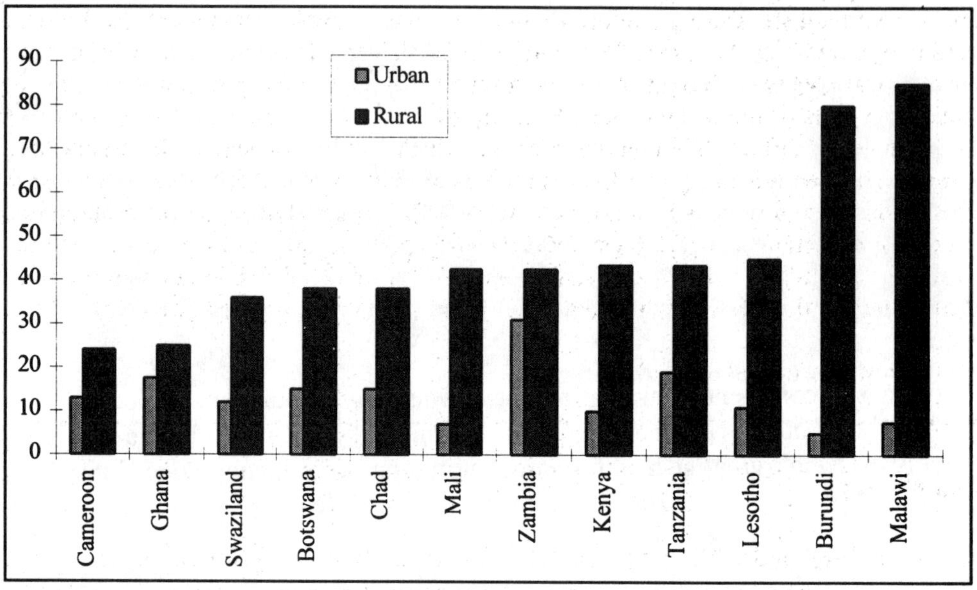

Source: World Bank 1996.

Poor parents (especially single female heads of households) are often overwhelmed by the daily burden of life and lack the time and resources to invest in their children, increasing the possibility that the intricate web of poverty will be intergenerationally spun to engulf their offspring as well. African women routinely perform multiple roles, supplying 70 percent of the labor for food production and heading between 25–50 percent of households in many countries while receiving only one-tenth of the continent's income (OAU and UNICEF 1992a). Attitudes towards girls' education and the household task burden of girls are fundamentally affected by this web of poverty as well.

At the same time that family income and purchasing power declined, governments in the region decreased their investment in the social sectors. Sub-Saharan Africa's public health and nutrition have been especially hard hit by reductions in the actual investment in the social sectors during the last decade. Evidence from UNICEF reports indicates that while the average percentage of government expenditure on education (12 percent) in SSA was slightly higher than that on defense, the average percentage of government expenditure on defense (9 percent) was more than twice that of health in 1994.

The absolute amount of expenditure on health and education was thus very little considering that the average GNP per capita was only about US $530 in 1992. In some countries, there has been a drastic reduction in the education budget as a percentage of government expenditure. Nigeria is one such example: in 1975, about 15 percent of government expenditure went to education, but this number decreased to less than 5 percent in 1990. In Ghana, cutbacks in pre-primary education particularly affected the poor (Box 1).

Box 1: The Demand for Child-Care in Poor Households

The participatory methods used in the Ghana Poverty Assessment revealed that childcare is a priority concern of poor mothers. During a priority ranking exercise, female members of the Asikuma Youth Association (generally aged between 25 and 40) who participated in the assessment identified a crèche as their principal concern. "Parents at Asikuma report that, under new government regulations, children under five years of age will no longer be accepted in state-run nurseries. This is likely to lead to a decline in the use of formal child minding services, which will be available in the private sector only. If this were to happen it is likely that larger numbers of mothers would either be compelled to stay at home or would have to carry their toddlers to work." The inquiry further revealed that pre-school is the part of the education spectrum most appreciated by poor households because of low opportunity costs (school-age children make significant contributions of labor and sometimes income in poor households) and for the release of the mother's or elder sibling's (most often girls) time.

Source: Andrew Norton and others 1994.

Population Growth

Between 1980 and 1992, while the world's population was growing at an average annual rate of 1.7 percent, Africa's population grew at 3.0 percent or nearly two-and-one-half times the world rate. It is projected that this rate will be maintained, or diminish only slightly well into the next decade, even as the other principal regions in the world are expected to experience dramatic declines in the overall population growth. In Zimbabwe, for example, where the population grew yearly at 3.13 percent for the past decade, it will double from 10 million to 20 million in the next 22 years.

Like a textbook case in demographic transition, Sub-Saharan Africa's high population growth rate stems from the rapid decline in mortality in recent years when fertility rates have remained, for the most part, at the same high levels that prevailed historically. For example, during the period, 1970–93, the crude death rate declined from 20 to 15 per 1,000 people. Yet fertility remains virtually unchanged with women averaging about 6 children per family. In fact, several traditional practices intended to ensure adequate spacing between children are rapidly giving way to modern lifestyles that have exacerbated the population problem. It is estimated that in 1993, there were a total of 541.5 million people in Sub-Saharan African. Out of these, about 20 percent (109 million) were children below 5 years of age and 47 percent were below 14 years of age. For example, in South Africa, children in the 0-14 year range make up 36.5 percent of the population (UNICEF 1993).

Sub-Saharan Africa today has the youngest population of any region in the world. This demographic explosion has disproportionately increased the number of children in the region seeking access to health services, food security, and education. While the OECD countries, given their rapidly aging structure, are shifting their attention to social security and gerontology, in the Sub-Saharan region, the focus is on social policy targeting young children. This is the case not only because they are the largest and fastest growing demographic group, but also because they face the highest current risks and their well-being will determine the future of these countries. Within a policy focused on the young, the development of more positive female gender roles is essential.

Figure 2: Population Age Structure in Sub-Saharan Africa

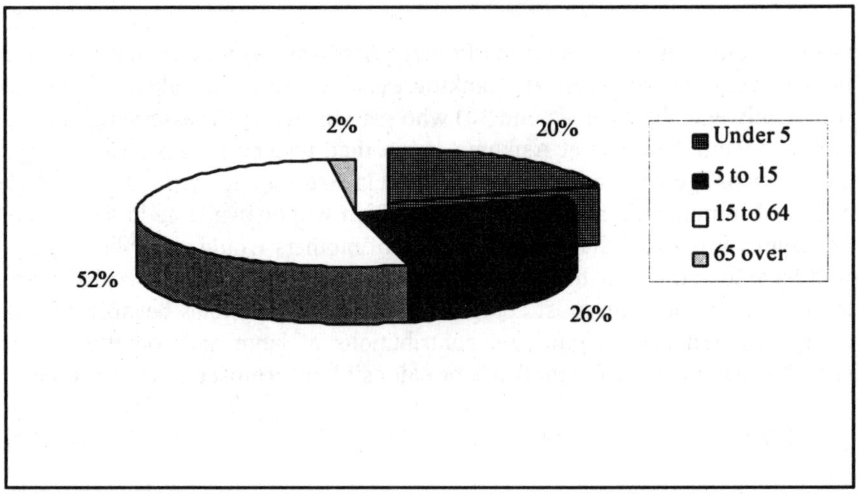

Sources: UNICEF 1995; World Bank 1995a.

Migration and Urbanization

Migration has combined with the already high natural population increase to cause accelerated urbanization in Sub-Saharan Africa, swelling its cities. The attraction of urban services and the search for better jobs in the wage-earning economy have motivated many people to leave their rural homelands. In scarcely a dozen years, the proportion of people living in cities increased from 23 per cent (1980) to almost 30 percent (1992), representing an average annual growth rate of 5 percent. At this rate, the urban population as a proportion of total population will have increased to 40 percent by the year 2000 . In many cities, the population is projected to double every 12 years.

These trends have significant implications for the health, care, and education of millions of young children. Rapid urbanization has caused large-scale unemployment and consequent urban poverty. For instance, it is estimated that Zimbabwe's unemployment rate in the formal sector was as high as 75 percent in 1992. Many live in overcrowded housing in slums with poor water and sanitary conditions leading to ill-health, especially among women and children. Poor sanitary conditions typically increase the domestic load of young girls who are typically responsible for fetching water (Box 2).

**Figure 3: Urban Population as A Percentage of Total Population
in Sub-Saharan Africa**

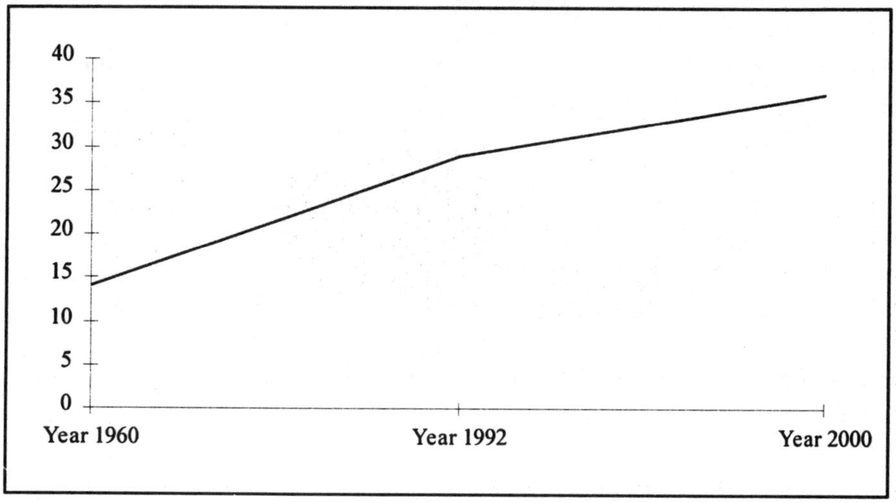

Source: UNDP 1994.

Changes in the Sub-Saharan African Family

As might be expected, the Sub-Saharan African family has not endured these changes unscathed. Because most rural-urban migrants are young men and women searching for better-paying jobs and independence, the urban age-pyramid is relatively young. In Ghana, there is evidence of girl-child labor migration without the accompanying parents. Many of the young migrants have children or, being of child-bearing age, will soon have them far away from the traditional support of extended families and relatives. In addition, while millions of men seek employment in urban areas and neighboring states, many wives have remained behind as single-parent heads of households, having to cope with multiple responsibilities of livelihood and child-care.

Box 2: Children in Poor Urban Households

The level of fertility amongst the urban poor may be viewed as an important element in the household survival strategy. Children and older members can be seen as resources to be used to allow those with the highest earning potential to maximize their income for the household's benefit. In Ghana, children's labor is typically used to support women's performance of a range of household and economic tasks. There are a number of activities that a household needs to perform that are not income-generating, especially in a context where there are considerable infrastructural deficiencies. The collecting of water, the obtaining of fuel, the disposal of refuse, queuing for services in conditions of overall scarcity - these tasks fall heavily upon the time-budgets of poor households. Whereas in the industrial world, children are viewed largely as domestic responsibilities, within the developing world, children are considered largely as domestic resources.

Source: Margaret Grieco and others 1994.

As a result, the African family structure has been experiencing changes that also contribute to the growing need for alternative forms of family support, child-care and early childhood development services. Extensive urbanization, labor migration, deterioration in rural conditions, unemployment, civil strife, and rapid social change all seriously threaten the traditional family structure. This emerging trend from extended to nuclear family (accompanied by an increasing number of female headed households and pregnant adolescents) is a prime contributor to the changing focus of child care in the Africa region.

One of the more dramatic developments in the African family structure is the increase in female-headed households, especially in rural areas. Although death and divorce frequently force women to head their households, male labor out-migration is the main cause of the rise in female-headed households in many of the African countries. It has been estimated that one-third of Sub-Saharan African households are now being headed by women. In Swaziland and Lesotho, nearly 60 percent of households are either headed by a woman or managed by a woman for much of the time. These women are not only responsible for the children and household chores, they must also work in the fields either cultivating subsistence crops or supplementing the family's cash income. Surveys show that the burden of child-care is increasingly falling on the elder female siblings who are often forced to drop out of school (Box 3).

**Box 3: Relationship between Girls' Secondary School Enrollment
and the Number of Pre-school Children in the Household**

The Kenya Participatory Poverty Assessment suggested that elder siblings (usually girls) were often prevented from attending school in order to take care of pre-school children in the household. This finding is confirmed by data from the *Kenya Welfare Monitoring Survey, 1994.*

No. of siblings aged 0-3 years	Net Secondary School Enrollment	
	Males	Females
0	18.9	20.6
1	13.3	13.7
More than 1	16.0	9.6

The data show that secondary school enrollment falls sharply for females when there is more than one child under four in the household. The impact of additional 4-6 year olds on secondary school enrollment was similar, although primary school enrollment did not appear to be so seriously influenced by the presence of younger siblings.

Source: World Bank and Government of Kenya 1994. Data analysis by Anil Deolalikar and Marito Garcia.

Whereas in some West African countries such as Nigeria, female-headed families are found to be wealthier than normal families because women are active in the trading business and have fewer dependents, in many others, women often continue to be excluded from investment in income-generating activities (trade, large farms, transportation or education for themselves and their children) and from access to basic productive assets of capital (credit) and land. They have lower levels of health, less food, poorer nutrition, and lower educational attainment, and can ill-afford child care. This has a profound negative impact on their children who are likely to remain trapped in a vicious cycle of deprivation and impoverishment. (World Bank 1992b).

Furthermore, new developments in the modern economy have encouraged women to join the labor market. The rate of female labor force participation in the wage-earning sector has become very high. From 1985 to 1990, the labor force participation rate of women in the 20-39 year range has gradually increased from 47.6 percent to 49 percent. As a result, an estimated 37 percent of the total labor force were women in 1990.

This expansion in female labor force participation has left increasingly more young children at home, poorly attended in the fields, or in the charge of their older siblings. In Kenya, for example, the commercialization of agriculture into tea and coffee plantations brought women into the labor force in large numbers, long hours spent in tea picking and reduced time for child-care (Box 4). To make matters worse, the traditional child-care support system that women once relied on has started to disappear as extended families become more difficult to sustain. From generation to generation, African societies had counted on the presence of an extended family for financial and emotional support in general, and child-care in particular. Children born into a warm, affectionate and welcoming culture, were sustained by a network of care and support that came from all extended family members. Though the hierarchical nature of this traditional child care system sometimes set limits to children's independence and mobility within the group, it provided them with security and acceptance demarcated by clearly-defined roles and relationships. The loss of this extended family involvement threatens the stability of the family, especially in the absence of other mechanisms to buttress the smooth cultural transmission of values and customs from grandparents to grandchildren.

Box 4: Portrait: A Tea-Plucker in Kericho

Tea-picker, mother of 1-year-old:

"I'm up by 4:30 a.m., make uji (porridge), after drinking, wash utensils, and get ready to pick tea, leaving at 6:30 a.m. After I leave, my older nursery school child takes care of the baby, including taking him with her to nursery school (carrying on back). The child taking most care of the baby is 9 years old. By 4:00 or 5:00 p.m., I am allowed to come home. I don't come home for lunch, since I prepare everything early in the morning, the 9-year-old can feed the baby during the day. After work, I look for vegetables and on Sundays I fetch firewood. While the vegetables are cooking I bathe, and by 6:00 p.m. I cook supper, so that we can eat and go to bed early - by 7:30 p.m. we are all in bed! The younger daughter washes.... When there is much tea to be picked, I come back late. I spend about 2 - 3 hours per day with my youngest children while we are awake."

Source: Swaedner 1994.

Another aspect of the changing face of the African family is adolescent pregnancy. For example, by age 18 more than 40 percent of the women in Côte d'Ivoire, Mali and Senegal have already given birth. Also, more and more of these pregnancies occur outside of wedlock. Research shows that early pregnancy is directly linked to increased pregnancy complications, higher maternal and infant mortality, as well as to less social and occupational mobility for both the mother and her child. The tendency for the children of teenage mothers to be more likely to become teenage mothers themselves has also been hypothesized. Without intervention, this vicious cycle of intergenerational dysfunctional socialization among poor parents in general, and teenage mothers in particular, will lead to a continuation of poverty and deprivation.

Changes in Child-Rearing Beliefs and Practices

The context of child-care in any society is composed of many things. Operating beside the socioeconomic climate just described, there are cultural, philosophical, and religious systems which constitute a base for the values and beliefs relevant to child-rearing. Parents have a set of child-rearing beliefs and practices that are derived from traditional culture and based on consensus within the culture about what is natural, normal, and necessary in raising young children (Levine and others 1994). Sub-Saharan Africa has long been classified as being at the traditional end of the modernization continuum. Child-rearing practices and beliefs are based largely on inherited and orally transmitted knowledge (Evans 1994). The context of child-care has been, until recently, rather stable and with adequate resources to support the traditional way of life. However, the invasion of modern-style concepts and changes in the economic conditions, social organization, and family structure -- such as the rise of female-headed households -- are reshaping, and in some instances even replacing, the traditional child-rearing beliefs and practices.

Although some traditional practices such as female circumcision have had deleterious effects on the African girl-child, many traditional child-rearing practices which have evolved over centuries have proven to be beneficial for children's optimal development. The replacement of these practices by 'modern' but inappropriate practices has had a negative impact on the healthy development of children. One prominent example of this is the change in attitudes toward breast-feeding. Traditionally, African mothers breast-fed their infants for a fairly extended period of time, a 'custom' which provides appropriate nutrition for the infant and also tends to improve the spacing between pregnancies. However, in the last decade, the promotion of infant formula has discouraged many mothers from breast feeding, mostly, but not exclusively in urban areas. One of the negative effects of the loss of such practices is reduced birth intervals (Box 5).

Box 5: Traditional Infant Care Practices in Africa

Anthropologists agree that African customs of infant care which include breast feeding on demand for 2 or 3 years , immediate attention to infant cries and other signals, frequent body contact and kinesthetic stimulation, begin with the goal of survival, although modern medicine has shown that certain practices such as the treatment of diarrhea with ritual healing are actually inimical to child health. The loss of one traditional practice - that of maintaining long birth intervals - has had serious consequences for both maternal and child health and overall development. Nothing was more characteristic of the African patterns of reproduction and infant care than a 24-40 month birth interval. This was accompanied by prolonged breast-feeding and maintained by post-partum sexual abstinence lasting as much as 2 years - an arrangement protected by polygynous marriage. A birth interval of at least two years was generally normative in rural communities, and women who bore children more often were socially stigmatized: When a woman breeds more rapidly people (in the Sukuma tribe of Tanzania) say "she gives birth like a chicken". Such customs which were universal in the region have eroded rapidly in the 20th century.

Source: Levine and others 1994.

Children in Crisis: Orphans, Refugees and the Displaced

UNICEF (1994) estimates that some 7-10 million households in Africa have had their livelihood wiped out by war and that an additional 5 million have been affected by drought or impoverished by apartheid. In addition, an estimated 5-10 million children become orphaned annually. Alternative care for these children bereft of material or moral support, will present a challenge of enormous proportions to Africa's scarce economic resources and institutional capacity. For physiological and social reasons, proper care for the orphaned teenage girl-children is especially important.

Civil conflicts and natural disasters in many parts of the African continent have led to the displacement of innocent people, many of whom are young children. There are an estimated 20 million refugees, with an average of 2,700 people per day being forced to leave their homelands and become refugees. In addition, about 18 million persons are considered internally-displaced (within their country of origin) and often do not qualify for international assistance as refugees (World Bank 1992a).

In 1989, Africa had the highest concentration of refugees/displaced persons in the world. A case in point is Mozambique where, between 1983 and 1991, more than 10 percent of the rural population fled to become refugees in neighboring countries and a further 25 percent were internally displaced. Today, UNICEF estimates that some 200,000 children are still either orphaned or separated from their families in Mozambique. In Malawi 1 out of 9.8 persons is a refugee, the highest among all the nations in the world (UNHCR 1993). In Liberia, nearly two-thirds of the population are currently displaced due to internal conflict. In Angola, about 10 percent of the population are displaced with an estimated 100,000 children separated from families or orphaned.

Of Africa's estimated 35 million refugees and displaced persons a disproportionate 80 percent are women and children (World Bank 1992a). For example, in Somali refugee camps in 1992, 60 percent were found to be children under 15 and 30 percent adult females. In addition, an increasing number of children, having lost their parents, are dislocated from their homes, and have become so-called 'street children.' Living in extreme material and social deprivation with little sense of safety and stability, the health and normal development of these children is severely hampered.

In sum, the alarming pace of economic decline, rapid population growth, increased urbanization, the changing family structure, and the increasing number of orphaned and displaced women and children from civil conflict and maternal catastrophes, have increased the likelihood that many Sub-Saharan African families must struggle in conditions of great adversity to care for, feed and educate their children. The situation of children in most Sub-Saharan African countries is clearly one of particularly high risk and is in need of urgent attention.

2. THE STATUS OF CHILDREN IN SUB-SAHARAN AFRICA[2]

Indicators of child welfare confirm that the adverse socioeconomic context just described has had a dramatic effect on child growth and development. Sub-Saharan Africa is the only major region in the world where the status of children has actually deteriorated in recent years.

This section begins with a brief discussion of SSA's human development condition as measured by the UNDP's Human Development Index (HDI). It then proceeds to describe the status of Sub-Saharan African children, including physical aspects such as survival, health, and nutrition, as well as educational and social-psychological aspects. For the convenience of description, the various types of physical, cognitive and socioemotional needs, and attendant indicators are separated. Yet it is important to note that they are operationally inseparable if we are concerned with fostering the healthy development of the whole child.

Progress in Human Development[3]

The Sub-Saharan Africa region lags significantly behind the rest of the developing world in human development, despite important gains over the past 30 years. The UNDP's Human Development Index (HDI) is a comprehensive measure of human development through combining indicators of real purchasing power, education and health. Using this indicator, the developing world has made clear progress in human development over the last three decades. Between 1960 and 1992, the overall HDI for developing countries increased from 0.26 to 0.54. Although the countries in SSA region also made progress, the region remains the least developed according to the HDI measurement. Forty-one of the 54 low human development countries are in Sub-Saharan Africa.

Physical Needs: Survival, Health, and Nutrition

An equal chance to survive is a basic right of all human beings. Yet Sub-Saharan Africa possesses the highest infant mortality rate in the world. Of the 40,000 children under the age of five who die in the world every day, over one-third are Africans, a proportion that is steadily rising. Sub-Saharan Africa accounts for only 12 percent of the world's population, but nearly 40 percent of child deaths. About 5 million child deaths occur in Sub-Saharan Africa each year. Within Sub-Saharan Africa, infant mortality rates range from a low of 47 per thousand in Zimbabwe to a high of 162 in Mozambique.

---

[2]   Within Sub-Saharan Africa region, there is a substantial amount of variation in child conditions and status. There is no such thing as an average African child. Efforts have been made throughout the report to give specific country examples.

[3]   This sub-section draws from World Bank 1994b.

Figure 4: UNDP Human Development Index

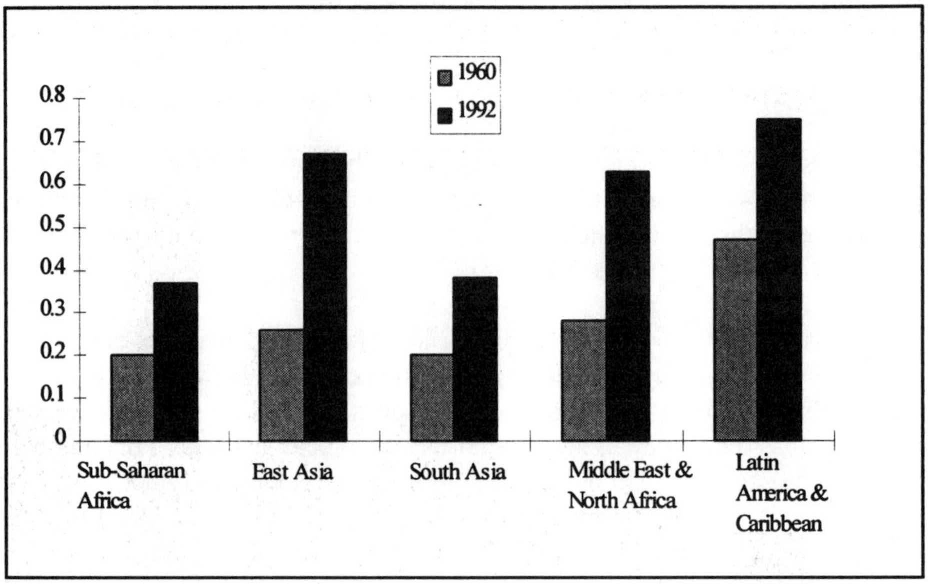

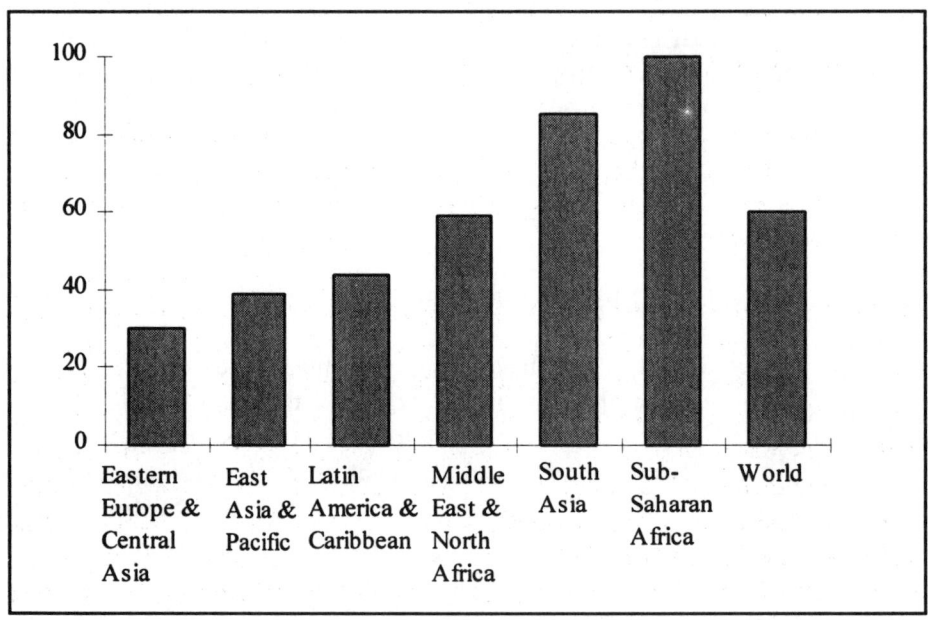

Source: UNDP 1994.

Figure 5: Infant Mortality Rate (per 1,000 live births)

Source: World Bank 1994a.

The under-5 mortality statistics indicate the probability that a newborn baby will die before reaching age 5. This shows the same pattern as that of infant mortality. In 1992, the regional odds of a child dying before the age of 5 were more than one in three (339 per thousand). The odds of early death are twice as high as the world average (173 per thousand) and over four times that of the European and Central Asian rate (75 per thousand). In Mozambique alone, more than half the children (552 out of per thousand) die before turning five.

Figure 6: Under-5 Mortality Rate 1992 (per 1,000 live births)

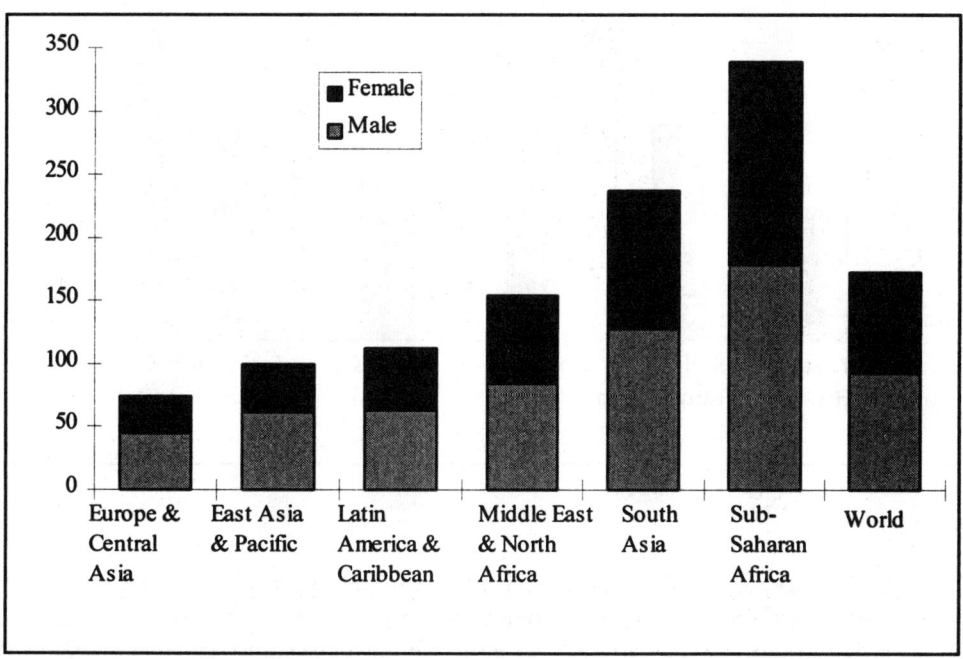

Source: World Bank 1994a.

Many of the same conditions of poverty and stress that place under 5 children at risk of death early in life, later leave them at risk of poor health, malnutrition, and impaired mental, social and emotional development. The absence of proper care and education in the early years have long-term consequences.

Regarding children's health status, although Sub-Saharan Africa has made significant progress, the health indices are still worse than those of any other region. The lack of clean water and safe sanitation are among the most critical determinants of good health. Only about 42 per cent of the Sub-Saharan population had access to safe water in 1993. This rate is the lowest among all the principal regions of the world and about half of the rate of the Arab States and Latin American countries (82 percent). Some countries are worse than others within the region. For instance, only one-tenth of the population in the Central Africa Republic had access to safe water in 1993. Access to sanitation and health services is also limited throughout Sub-Saharan Africa. In 1993, only 26 percent of the population had adequate sanitation, and about 56 percent could count on health services. Without safe water and adequate sanitation, fly-transmitted diseases are dominant in the heat, particularly in urban slum areas. In rural areas, millions of women and children must walk a long distance just to fetch a jar of water. This lack of drinking water locally adds to the already high transport burden for women and children, who are responsible for over 70 percent of transport in terms of time and over 80 percent in terms of effort (Urasa 1990).

**Figure 7: Percent of Population With Access to Health Services,
Safe Water, and Sanitation**

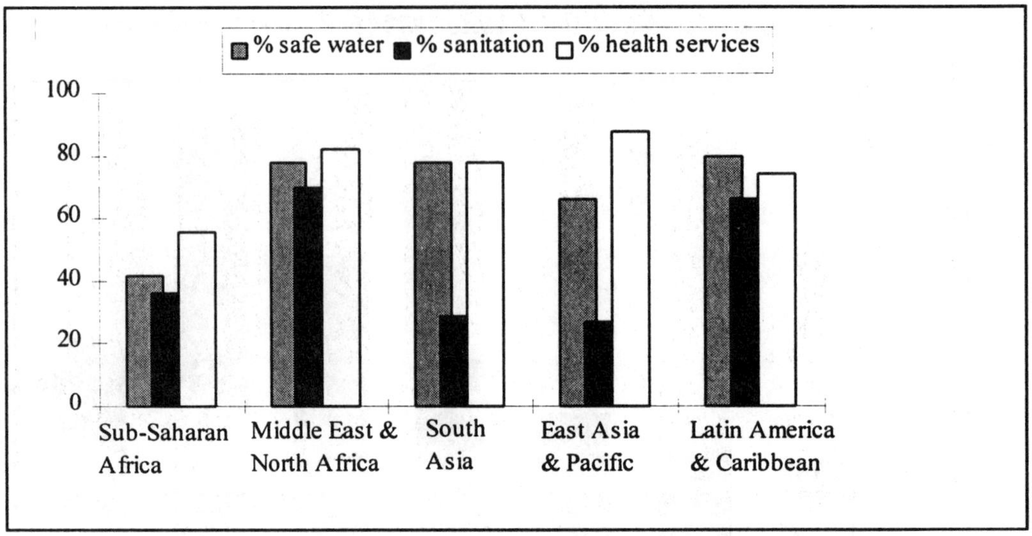

Source: UNICEF 1995.

In 1991, only 63 percent of the children in the region had been immunized against tuberculosis and less than 50 percent against DPT (diphtheria, pertussis, and tetanus), polio and measles. This is far short of the 90 percent goal for the year 2000 set at the World Summit for Children. Only 46 percent of children under five have access to oral rehydration therapy (World Bank 1995a). These numbers are strikingly low in comparison to what has been achieved in other developing regions: 94 percent in East Asia and the Pacific, 86 percent in South Asia, 87 percent in the Arab states, and almost 80 percent in Latin America and Caribbean region.

Malnutrition is widespread in Sub-Saharan Africa. Sixteen percent of the babies born in Sub-Saharan Africa in 1992 suffered from low birth weight, compared to seven percent among highly developed countries (UNDP 1994). Low birth weight, defined as babies who are born weighing less than 2,500 grams, is associated with poor maternal health and malnutrition, and tends to lead to poor growth in infancy and childhood. The proportion of low birth weight babies in the region ranges from a low of 8 percent in Botswana to a high of 21 percent in Burkina Faso.

About 29 million children (30 percent) of the under-5 population are underweight. Children under the age of 5 are considered underweight if they weigh-in at two standard deviations below the median weight for age of the reference population. This rate is almost three times that of the Latin America and Caribbean area and four times that in industrial countries. Within Sub-Saharan Africa, the prevalence of underweight children varies substantially. It ranges from a low of 12 percent in Côte d'Ivoire to as high as 49 percent in Niger, Tanzania, and Mauritania. About 12 countries in Sub-Saharan Africa have an underweight rate exceeding 25 percent.

Figure 8: Percent of 1-year-olds immunized against TB, DPT, and Measles

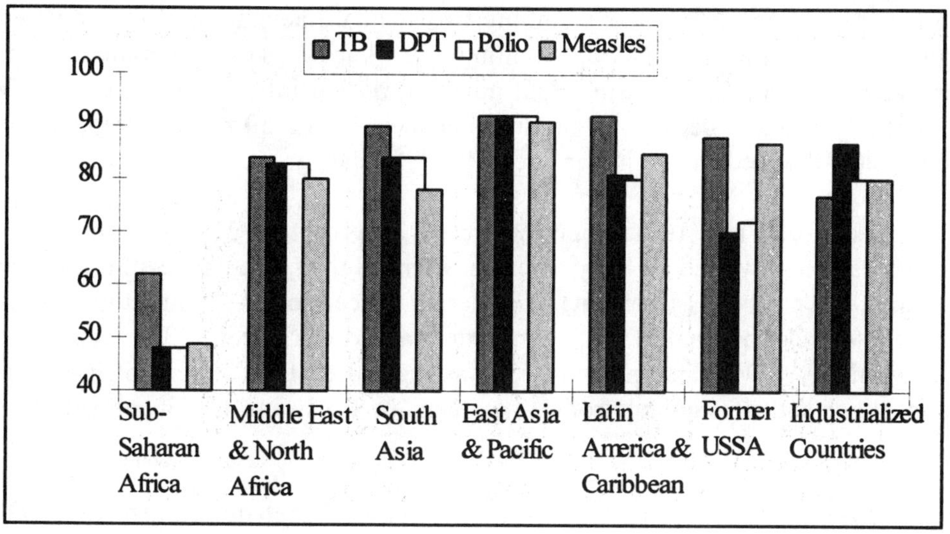

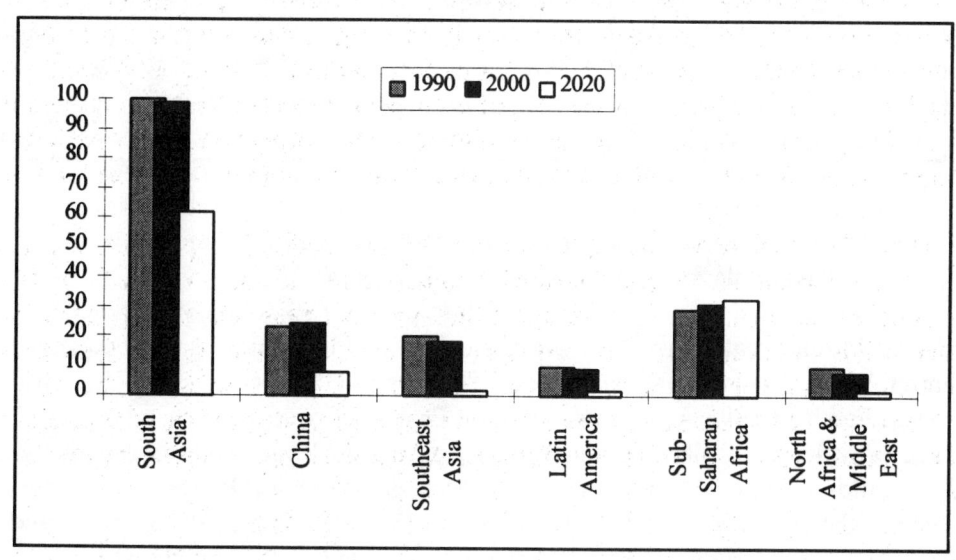

Source: UNICEF 1995.

By the year 2020, virtually each region in the world will experience a reduction in the absolute numbers of underweight pre-school children, with the notable exception of Sub-Saharan Africa. Even an optimistic scenario puts the number of malnourished at about 34 million in the year 2020. Unless the population growth rates (currently at 3 percent) are dramatically reduced, the absolute number of underweight children will rise even if the prevalence rates are kept at present levels in 2020 (Garcia 1994).

Figure 9: Projections of Numbers of Underweight Pre-school Children (millions), by Region, Optimistic Scenario, 2020

Source: M. Garcia 1994.

Two other indicators associated with malnutrition are 'wasting' and 'stunting.' 'Wasting', or acute malnutrition, refers to the situation where emergencies such as sickness or food shortage cause the child to become underweight relative to height. It is medically defined as children between 12 and 23 months weighing two standard deviations below the median weight for height of the reference population. 'Stunting', also known as chronic malnutrition, refers to a situation where a child, due to insufficient nutrition during infancy, becomes abnormally short relative to age, medically defined as children between 24 and 59 months standing two standard deviations below the median height-for-age of the reference group.

Between 1980 and 1991, approximately 12 percent of 12 to 23 month-olds in Sub-Saharan Africa were 'wasted.' This proportion is more than three times the incidence in Latin America and the Caribbean (4 percent). Another 42 percent of 24–59 months olds are 'stunted.' Again, this rate is double that of the Latin America and Caribbean (23 percent) region (World Bank 1993; UNDP 1994). The incidence of wasting varied from 2 percent in Zimbabwe to 23 percent in Niger and of stunting from 14 percent in Botswana to 43 percent in Nigeria and Malawi.

Figure 10: Percent of Children Underweight, Wasted, and Stunted, 1991

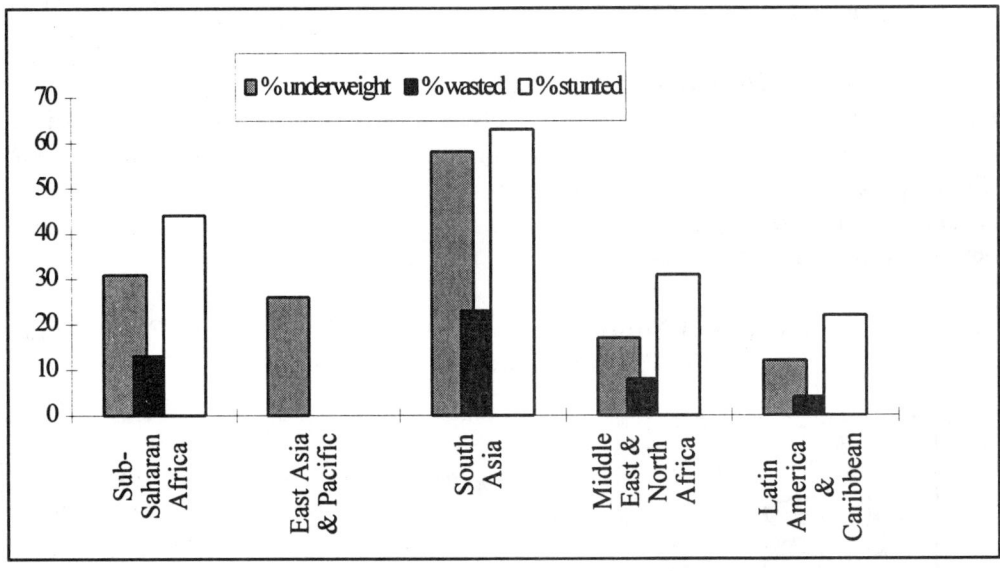

Source: UNICEF 1995.
Note: Information on proportion children wasted and stunted not
       available for East Asia and Pacific region

Malnutrition greatly increases the risk of morbidity which is correspondingly high in Sub-Saharan Africa. Demographic and Health Surveys (DHS) conducted by the Africa Regional Nutrition and Family Health Analytical Initiative Project between the period 1986–92, show that the average prevalence of diarrhea among children under 2 years is 34 percent. About 1 in 2 Senegalese children under 24 months had diarrhea in the 2 weeks preceding the survey, the highest among the countries surveyed. Most deaths from diarrhea could be prevented by almost cost-free oral rehydration therapy (ORT) and continued feeding. Thirty-six percent were reported to have had a bad fever, and another 31 percent were found to have had a cough or suffered from rapid breathing. Both are major causes of pneumonia, death from which could be prevented by the early prescription of low-cost antibiotics. Other indirect effects of malnutrition include delayed mental development and enrollment in school (Box 6).

A new and further threat to the health status of mothers and children in Sub-Saharan Africa is AIDS. This human immunodeficiency virus is now a formidable threat to Africa's health as well as to its social and economic well-being. In 1992, approximately 6.5 million people were infected by HIV in Sub-Saharan Africa and two-thirds of all new cases are occurring on the continent. With increasing numbers of HIV-infected mothers giving birth to infected children, Africa is being robbed of both its present and its future. An estimated 1 million (14 percent) of the total HIV-infected people are children, and this number may increase to 2 million by the end of this century.

Box 6: Malnutrition and Delayed Primary School Enrollment

A World Bank paper investigated why children in low income countries often delay primary school enrollment despite the prediction of human capital theory that schooling will begin at the earliest possible age. The study explored a number of explanations for delayed enrollment and tested alternative hypotheses using data from a household survey in Ghana. The estimates, which address a number of previously-ignored econometric issues, strongly support the notion that childhood malnutrition causes delayed enrollment*. A Participatory Poverty Assessment in Tanzania shows how delayed enrollment can be particularly detrimental to girls' education. It drastically reduces the number of years a girl spends in school as she is usually forced to drop out at puberty.

*The delays can be caused by illnesses or the perception of parents and teachers that the child is not ready for school.

Source: Glewwe and Jacoby 1992.

Infant mortality rates may be at least 30 percent higher than they would have been in the absence of AIDS, and many children will survive only to enter a more precarious environment upon a parent's death from AIDS. Children who lose their parents to AIDS are often forced to drop out of school to survive. In Tanzania, for instance, the widespread prevalence of AIDS is associated with the withdrawal of girls from school and with marriage at an early age, eroding much of the progress made in female education (Ainsworth and others 1992; Shaeffer 1993).

In sum, a significant proportion of Sub-Saharan African children live in poor health, are malnourished and have either fallen prey or are vulnerable to infectious diseases. Even short-term nutritional deprivation in the early years of life can lead to long-term damage, thus influencing the capacity to learn and grow, and later influencing adult productive capacity. Poverty and lack of information are the main causes of malnutrition and disease. Interventions such as early detection by monitoring growth in childhood and during pregnancy, food supplementation, nutrition and health education, and medical referral of malnourished /sick children contribute to the reduction of child mortality and malnutrition.

Educational Profile

Education is a critical determinant of the well-being of future generations, especially for females, because it contributes to future potential income and can improve parental child-rearing practices. Empirically, this lesson emerges from Asia where rising investments in the 1960s and 1970s in education established the human capital for the economic growth that followed (World Bank 1995c).

The Universal Declaration of Human Rights states that "everyone has a right to education." In addition to the basic physical needs such as food, health and shelter, children also have strong innate needs to learn and acquire skills, knowledge, attitudes, and habits that foster personal development. To fully develop their potential as members of society, or simply as human beings, these needs have to be satisfied in a stimulating and caring environment. How do Sub-Saharan African children fare in this regard?

Sub-Saharan Africa is caught in an educational downward spiral. Despite the unprecedented expansion in education in the post-colonial period, Africa remains the most under educated continent in the world. The proportion of the population over age 15 who cannot, with comprehension, read and write a short, simple, statement of their everyday life was 50 percent in 1990 (figure 11). This makes Africa's adult illiteracy rate second only to South Asia's and about three times greater than that of Latin America and the Caribbean (18 percent) (World Bank 1994a). As much as 82 percent of the population in Burkina Faso remained illiterate in the year 1990. In Malawi, only 38 percent of the population was literate in 1994. Of particular relevance is the high rate of illiteracy among women. Two out of 3 women in Sub-Saharan Africa are illiterate (62 percent). In 9 out of 47 Sub-Saharan Africa countries, female illiteracy rates exceed 80 percent. In Burkina Faso 91 percent of the female population was illiterate in 1992.

The mean years of schooling for Sub-Saharan Africa was only 1.6 in 1992 (figure 12), the lowest among all the developing regions in the world. This has placed the Sub-Saharan Africa region at a great disadvantage at the outset of the globalized economy and information age where competition requires not only literacy in terms of reading and writing, but also coping with modern technology.

Figure 11: Illiteracy Rate, 1990

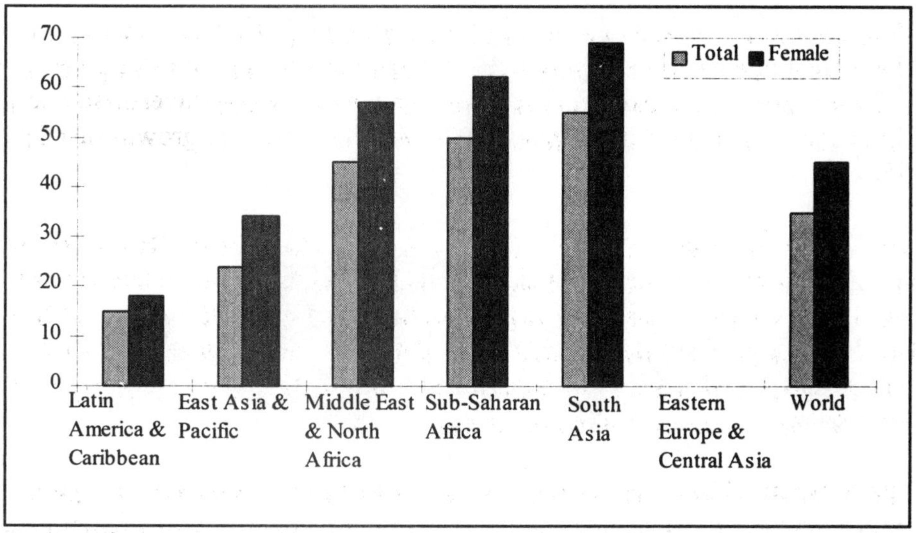

Source: World Bank 1994a.[4]

The mean years of schooling for women in the region is only 1.0, compared to 2.2 for men (Odaga and Heneveld 1995). These statistics are significant in view of the recognized relationship between women's education and the improved health status and educational attainment of their offspring. Accumulated research evidence suggests that a mother with a few years of schooling is more likely to provide her children with the care, stimulation and nutrition which will dramatically improve her child's educational participation and performance in the early formative years, than a mother who has never been in school. In Africa, an increase of 1 percentage point in the national literacy rate is directly associated with a 2 year rise in life expectancy (Cochrane, as cited in Lockheed and Verspoor 1990).

The education profile of African children is characterized by low enrollment and high attrition in primary schools and the poor participation in secondary and tertiary levels. Regionally, the expansion of primary enrollment during the 1960s and 1970s gave way to stagnation and even decline during the last decade. The present low primary enrollment levels and high repetition and drop-out rates in many Sub-Saharan countries are in large part due to poor investment in children before entry. This is compounded by poor quality and low efficiency in the existing primary school systems.

---

4   No figures were available for Eastern Europe & Central Asia.

Figure 12: Mean Years of Schooling

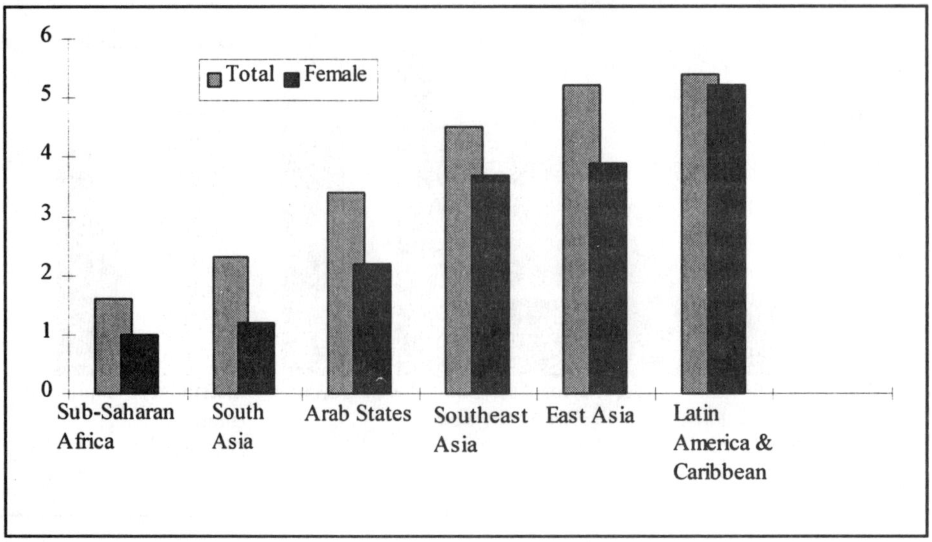

Source: UNDP 1994.

The gross enrollment ratios (GER)—the proportion of pupils of all ages in primary education to the total official primary school-age population—indicate that the Sub-Saharan Africa region lags considerably behind others. During the period 1986–92, the Sub-Saharan African average GER was only 74 percent for males and 60 percent for females. Many girl children have high task-loads at home and in the fields, and are consequently being withheld from school. At the same time, the industrial countries averaged about 102 percent for both boys and girls (UNICEF 1995). These regional averages conceal some very poor performers: the GER in Mali was only 25 percent, and in Somalia 11 percent, the lowest in the world (UNESCO 1992). No fewer than 18 countries in Sub-Saharan Africa reported declining GERs throughout the last decade.

Figure 13: Gross Enrollment Ratio

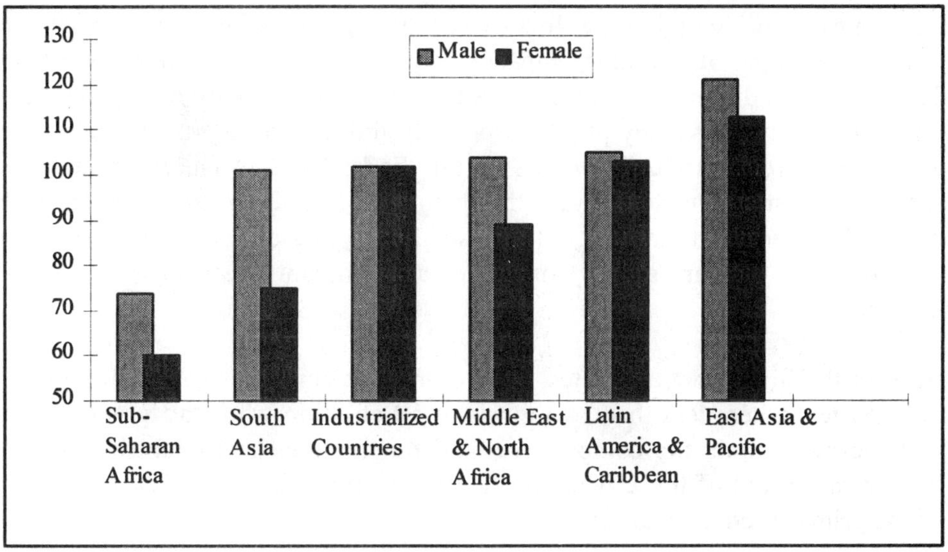

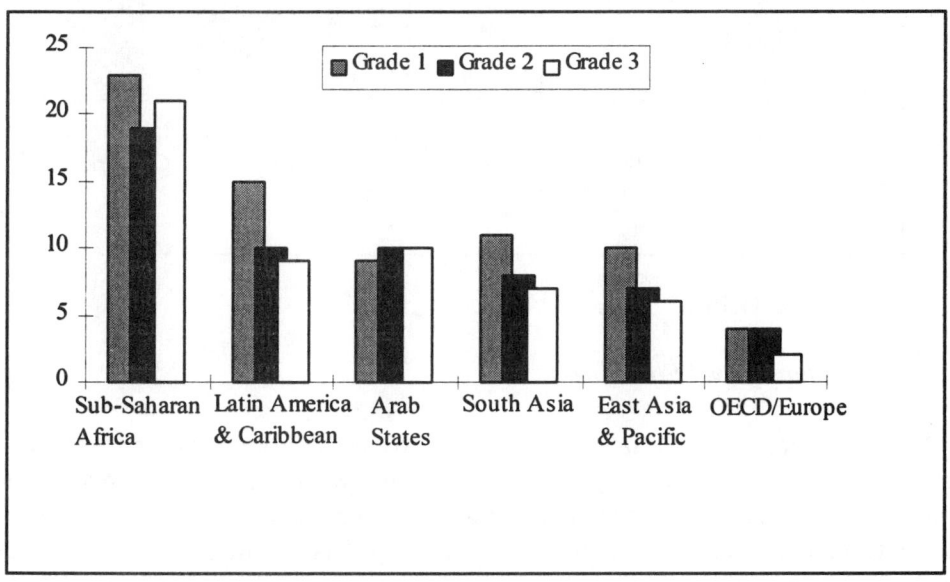

Source: UNICEF 1995.

About 50 percent of the total primary school-aged population in Sub-Saharan Africa are out of school. If current trends continue, the absolute number of children excluded from primary school will rise to 52 million by the turn of the century (UNESCO 1993). In Uganda, for example, out of 3.5 million children of primary school age (6-12), only 1.9 million were actually in school in 1994. Most of these out of school children live in urban slums or in rural areas, assisting in the fields or herding livestock.

Figure 14: Repetition Rates in Grades 1–3 in Primary Education

Source: UNESCO 1992.

For those who do enroll, the existing primary school system in Sub-Saharan Africa is plagued by poor quality and low internal efficiency. While repetition rates are very high in all grades, they are particularly high in the first two or three grades where the admission of children from a wide age-range of learning capacity typically leads to overcrowded classrooms, unsuitable learning conditions, demotivating teaching practices, and subsequent early dropout. Evidence has shown that for many pupils, especially those from deprived family backgrounds, repeating one or more unproductive years at this early stage of their formal education can constitute the first destructive step toward dropping out. Twenty or more percent of children in Sub-Saharan Africa repeat at least 1 grade between the years of 1 to 3 (UNESCO 1993). This high repetition rate in primary school constitutes a significant waste of Africa's financial and human resources.

Besides the high repetition rates, school dropout continues to be a major problem for Sub-Saharan Africa, where less than two-thirds of all children who start grade 1 actually reach grade 5. At the same time, the comparative statistic for industrial countries is more than 95 percent. For instance, out of those who enrolled in primary school in Uganda, only 32 percent completed the primary school cycle in 1994.

Figure 15: Percent of Primary School Entrants Reaching Grade 5

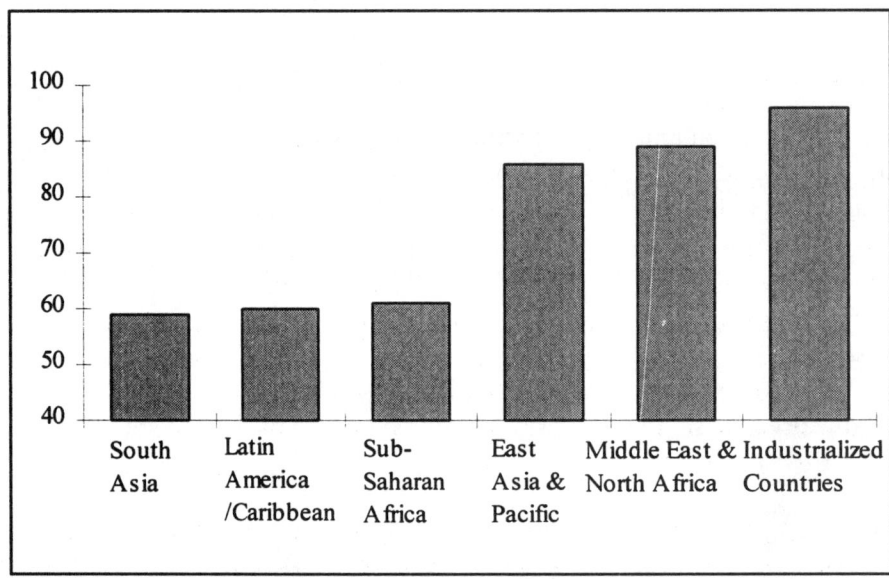

Source: UNICEF 1995.

Secondary and Tertiary Level Enrollment

Only 18 percent of those falling within the official age-brackets for secondary education were actually enrolled in secondary education in the year 1991, the lowest among all the developing regions including South Asia. Female secondary enrollment is an even lower at 14 percent. Inadequate preparation in primary schooling has resulted in even higher rates of repetition and dropout at the secondary level.

Figure 16: Secondary School Enrollment

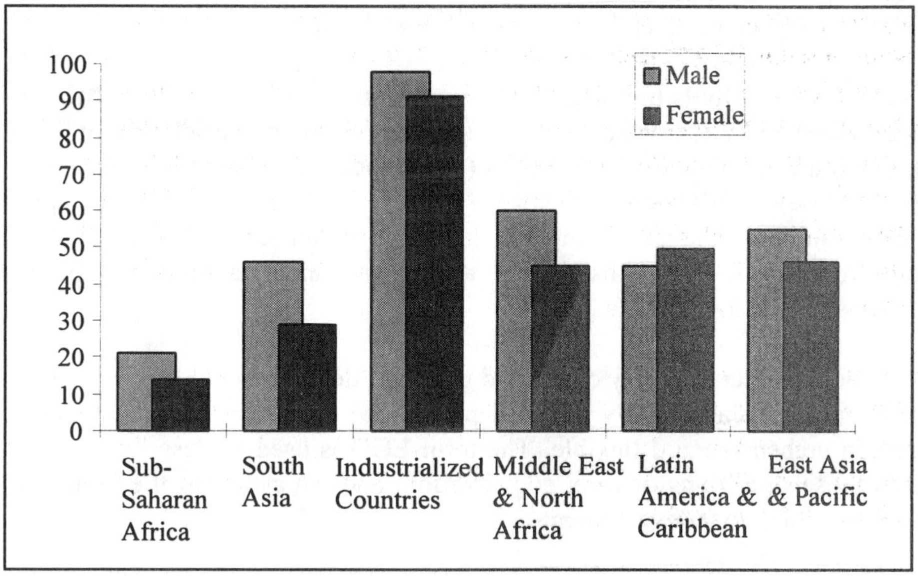

Source: UNICEF 1995.

Early Interventions, School Readiness and Subsequent Performance

One of the key factors contributing to primary school inefficiency is that most of the African children are not adequately prepared for schooling when they enter the first grade. Many of them enter the school system malnourished from inadequate food intake, weakened by illnesses and having received little cognitive stimulation as toddlers. Little or no attention has been paid to early developmental needs, especially in poor households. Child quality, those characteristics the learner brings to the classroom that play a significant role in determining school outcomes, is not ensured. The inadequacy of *school readiness* is reflected not in a child's lack of knowledge about letters and numbers, nor in basic school-related skills such as following instructions or sitting still, but more important, in the capacity of the child to process and respond to stimuli.

When a child gets proper nutrition, health care, and stimulation during the preschool years, the quality of the child sitting in the classroom improves, *Active Learning Capacity* (ACL)—or propensity and ability to interact with and take optimal advantage of the full complement of resources offered by any formal or informal learning environment—improves. Thus the efficiency of learning improves (Levinger 1994, 1995). However, children in Sub-Saharan Africa are plagued by poor nutrition and inadequate health practices resulting in inadequate ALC for primary schooling. In addition, the heavy work-load at home, especially on girl-children, has resulted in high rates of absenteeism from school. The poor quality of schooling has already been mentioned.

The Challenge Ahead

These aggregate statistics sketch a bleak picture of the African child. However, one important source for optimism is the high value placed on children in households all over the

African continent. Children, to Africans are the "essence or sap of life," and according to a Yoruba folk song are essential "adornments" for parents. It should be possible to build on this basic motivation for promoting child welfare and development.

The first step towards building a genuine commitment to improving the status of young children is to increase the aggregate resources spent on children, particularly in the 0-8 years old period. This will mean a threefold strategy of (a) reallocating existing spending away from non-productive (defense) to productive sectors; (b) improving income raising capacity; and (c) involving communities in the management and support of their children's development. The next step is to introduce ways to enhance the awareness, understanding and practice of early childhood care and development (ECD).

What do we mean by early childhood care and development? Many people misinterpret it to mean merely an academically oriented pre-school education. In fact, ECD programs are much more comprehensive and flexible. The term ECD is used to describe a range of services that promote those conditions of care, socialization, and education in the home or community that enhances a child's total development.

ECD programs can happen in a variety of settings such as a school site, a family home, a church, through the mass media, or even informal gatherings. Several channels can be used to improve child development, beginning with parents themselves and other caregivers, who can be provided with information and training. Some services can be delivered directly to children, whereas others can be provided indirectly, by promoting community development as a basis for the social and political change required to improve conditions that affect child development, by increasing public awareness of and demand for early childhood services, and by strengthening the institutions that provide them. Non-formal channels have proved affordable and effective (Psacharopoulos 1995).

The type of programs best suited to this purpose vary according to the age-group concerned and the comprehensiveness of services provided, including health, nutrition, and developmentally appropriate learning contexts. There is a risk of inappropriate combinations such as relegating the custodial care of 0-3 years olds to institutional settings planned for 4-5 years olds using models of instruction designed for 6–8 years olds (Woodhead 1995). How a child's developmental needs can and should be satisfied vary according to the particular characteristics of his or her environment (Asomaning and others 1994).

Within this 'holistic' ECD approach, a dual strategy is often pursued which seeks to raise child quality and increase the effectiveness of parenting through the involvement of local communities. ECD programs provide appropriate care which addresses the physical, cognitive, social and emotional needs of children. It prepares them for entry into school and subsequent life in multiple reinforcing ways including adequate nutrition, good health, sufficient cognitive stimulation and care so that their active learning capacity and wherewithal for social integration are maximized.

3. WHAT CAN EARLY CHILDHOOD DEVELOPMENT PROGRAMS DO?[5]

A growing body of global evidence has emerged that supports the case for early childhood care and development programs. In general, research focusing on the effects of ECD programs on children's development concludes that these programs promote the well-being of the whole child. In particular, they foster language, cognitive, and social development through frequent and varied verbal interaction, and provision of educational curricula that permit children to initiate and pace their own learning activities and opportunities to interact with adults and peers (e.g. Darlington and others 1980; Hayes and others 1991).

While evidence from Africa is still lacking, research done in other parts of the world, especially in the US and Latin America, has demonstrated that the effects of ECD programs are especially beneficial for children from poor families not capable of providing a healthy, safe and stimulating environment for children. Intensive exposure to a well-planned child care intervention project, particularly one that serves both child and family, and provides integrated services in health, nutrition and education can improve the lives of these children and have important positive implications for intellectual development and later school and social adaptation. In the US, research on the effects of the national Head Start program which serves poor children found evidence of its positive effects on IQ, on developed abilities at point of entry into school, and on achievement at the end of early grades (Hubbell and others 1985). As described in the previous sections, most of the Sub-Saharan children fit into this category of at risk population.

The following section summarizes the potential benefits and rationale for investment in programs of early childhood care and development in the Sub-Saharan Africa region.

Improving Child Quality

How individuals function in their life hinges, to a significant extent, on experiences during their first few years. This claim is substantiated by research evidence which shows that human brain development takes place most rapidly during infancy and early childhood. These years are critical in the formation and development of intelligence, personality, and social behavior. By age 6, for example, a child's brain has reached 90 percent of its adult size. During these initial years, therefore, all children have a particular need for love and care, sufficient nutrition, and stimulation and encouragement to develop all their brain faculties. Intervention at this time will yield the maximum benefits. The special supplemental nutrition program for women, infants, and children (WIC) in the US has helped reduce fetal death rate by 20–33 percent; increased the head size of infants, and result in better vocabulary test scores among 4- and 5-year-olds whose mothers had participated when pregnant.

Many Sub-Saharan African families are unable to provide children with adequate nutrition, a safe and healthy physical environment, and stimulation for the developing brain and

---

[5]   This section draws heavily from Myers 1992a and Young 1995.

mind. This results in a child's inability to take full advantage of schooling. Because of the importance of the early formative years, elementary schooling and even kindergarten may be too late to develop these capacities in children. Early childhood development programs are needed to support parents by providing their children the ingredients necessary for healthy development.

Increasing the Efficiency of Primary and Secondary School Investments

Early childhood development programs can increase the efficiency, reduce the cost and thus raise the return to primary and secondary school investment, by increasing access to primary education, lowering the repetition and drop-out rates and improving the quality of learning. ECD programs can facilitate increased primary school attendance directly by enabling older siblings to go to school. These children often have to drop out of school to act as care-givers for younger children if not for the provision of ECD programs. A study conducted in Brazil in 1980 (and the Kenyan data cited in Box 3) concluded that the number of younger siblings age 0–6 have a highly significant negative effect on the school attendance for children age 7–14 (Psacharopoulos and Arriagada 1989). ECD programs also raise awareness of the importance of education within the community and thus tend to further increase the primary enrollment level.

As mentioned previously, ECD programs can increase child quality and enhance learning readiness upon entry into primary school. When children have a higher active learning capacity upon entry into primary school, they can make better use of the school. Consequently, the efficiency of primary and secondary school will be increased. Empirical evidence from Myers (1992b) review of nineteen longitudinal evaluations examining the effect of early interventions in Latin America reveals that children who participated in early childhood programs experience lower repetition rates in primary school. The beneficial impact of early education is particularly pronounced among girls and children from rural, indigenous, and lower-level socioeconomic backgrounds. A two pronged approach to improve the environment in lower primary school is likely to be even more effective in improving primary school outcomes.

Enhancing the Economic Contribution of the Child to Society

Early childhood development programs improve children's physical and mental capacity. Over the long term, this can result in higher productivity and cost savings associated with better health and development. ECD programs affect enrollment, progress, and performance in schooling which is associated with effectiveness of education. By reducing repetition rates the external impact of classroom crowding is reduced, improving school quality. Besides improving the efficiency of educational systems, early childhood education also helps reduce costs in other social areas such as preventing deviant behavior and crimes, thus cutting the later need for social welfare programs and lowering spending on corrective measures. Empirical evidence of the economic return to early childhood education was established by the High Scope Perry Preschool study in the US, a program of early intervention for low-income children who were at risk of school failure. Between 1962 and 1967, 56 children, age 3-4 from Michigan, received 2 years of pre-school education (2.5 hours per day) coupled with weekly home visits. Information on participants, and a control group, was collected annually while the children were between years 3-11 and again at ages 14, 15, and 27.

One-third more of the high scope children graduated from regular or adult high school (71 percent vs. 54 percent). At age 27, four times as many program members as control ones earned $2,000 or more per month (29 percent vs. 7 percent). The proportion of non-participants arrested were five times greater than that of the participants (35 percent vs. 7 percent). A cost-benefit analysis was conducted by estimating the monetary value of the program and its effects, in constant 1992 dollars discounted annually at 3 percent. Dividing the $88,433 in benefits per participant by the $12, 356 in cost per participant results in a benefit-cost ratio of 7.16 returned to the public for every dollar invested in the High/Scope Perry program (Schweinhart and others 1993).

Reducing Social Inequity

Evidence suggest that investing in human capital, especially in early development, also attacks some of the most intractable causes of poverty. A large part of cognitive achievement differentials between lower and higher socioeconomic groups can be attributed to the malnutrition, poor health due to the lack of sanitation, and low levels of psychological stimulation in childhood. All of these factors can be positively affected by education. Early child development interventions can help reduce social inequalities rooted in poverty by helping to provide young children from disadvantaged backgrounds with a more equitable or 'fair' start in life and a foundation for further schooling. ECD programs can help compensate for historic inequities transmitted intergenerationally in poor households.

In South Africa, for example, the average monthly household income for whites in 1991 was R4679, (US $1023) more than four times larger than that of the black African households. Studies show that within the education systems for black Africans, repetition and drop-out rates contrast sharply with statistics from the education systems for whites. One recent study shows that white people are seven times more likely to be literate than the black in South Africa (Fuller and others 1995). Early childhood programs are essential to help reduce such stark inequity between black and white Africans by providing disadvantaged children with proper health care, nutrition, and education, which their families are not able to provide. South Africa has recognized the importance of early intervention by making a "reception year" for 5-year olds a major point of their new education policy (African National Congress 1994). One of the new priorities for Social Welfare Policy is vulnerable children under 5 years of age. The "Flagship Program for unemployed women with 0-5 year olds" launched in 1996 will pilot programs which may be replicable on a larger scale (Box 7).

The advantages of early childhood intervention are especially apparent for girls. Differential treatment of girls begins early in many of the African cultures—female primary enrollment rates, for example, are less than 50 percent of those of boys in many Sub-Saharan African countries. Strategies to improve girls' participation include scholarships as well as attention to their readiness for primary school. Early childhood programs can be an important aid in helping to overcome discriminatory barriers and gender inequalities that already exist at the time of first entry into school.

Four issues emerge which require careful consideration in balancing center-based with home-based and other alternative delivery systems, e.g. health centers, women's organizations and extension systems. They are: (a) the large numbers and related unit costs involved in service delivery; (b) the ability to pay among the poor and most needy; (c) the quality of service; and (d) the effects of training and certification on differentiating, and sometimes discrediting, home-based care-givers from center-based workers. What is needed is a standards policy based on performance standards negotiated by all stakeholders. Such a process acknowledges prior learning and experience and non-formal training, while ensuring quality of care. Such particular issues, and the many others explicitly or implicitly raised in this paper, will certainly contribute to the growing ECD research agenda for Africa.

Box 7: What does the Literature from South Africa Suggest ?

A longitudinal study conducted in South Africa by Short and Biersteker (1984), followed lower-class children who participated in the pre-school program developed by the Early Learning Resource Unit (ELRU).

The study focused on the scholastic progress of children who attended the Athlone Early Learning Centre (ELC) between January 1972 and December 1974. Besides those attending the ELC, there were three other groups of children included in the study. These were 1) an 'unschooled' lower-class group from the same population as those attending the ELC; 2) a more middle-class group of children attending a pre-school in the same home ownership section of Athlone; and 3) a group of lower-class children from another township, also attending a preschool. The children from the ELC and the control group children were followed for 12 years. The study was done in 3 phases. Phase 1 consisted of the data collected on the children while they were in the preschool (1972--74). The second phase assessed children during the first year of primary school, with a focus on psychosocial behavior and language ability (1973–75.) In addition, school performance data were collected on the children through 1980. The third phase was undertaken in 1983-1984, when the children were in high school.

The results indicated that children who participated in the ELC program performed like the more middle-class children as a result of their preschool program, compensating for social class differences. From the phase 1 study the authors concluded that: the ELC program helped to overcome the effects of disadvantaged socio-economic backgrounds, ensuring a basic level of school readiness (1984:23). Further, they concluded that as a group:

Ex-ELC (Early Learning Centre) pupils . . . were more likely to show 'creative inquisitiveness,' academic motivation, good socio-emotional adjustment and rapid adjustment to primary school than children from the same community who had not attended a preschool programme.

In the phase II tests, those who attended the ELC did better than non-preschool children suggests the robustness of the impact of the pre-school experience.

Phase 3, the longitudinal follow-up of the children focused on their scholastic achievement. This was a simple measurement of grade level achieved. What is remarkable is that it was possible to follow 88.2 percent of the original ELC sample. Unfortunately, the comparison group had far more attrition and, thus, the researchers felt there was no adequate group against which to compare the ELC children. What they chose to do was to compare the ELC children with national cohort data.

What were the results? The drop-out rates were reduced. All the ex-ELC pupils remained at school to age 12, by age 15, 95.2 percent were still in school and by age 17, 68.2 percent were still in school (1984:106). The comparable data for the national cohort would suggest the same rate of attendance at age 12, but significant differences occur at age 15 when only 57.8 percent are still in school; at age 17 there are only 18.1 percent in school (1984:73); thus, those who attended pre-school were more likely to remain in school for a longer period of time than their peers who did not have a pre-school experience.

continued on page 31)

(continued from page 30)

Another hypothesized effect of pre-school education is a decrease in the repetition rate. Repetition rates, as calculated by the percentage of children who are on-grade for their age, were high for the total sample. However, they were lower for the ELC group than the national cohort. In the study sample, 67 percent of the 12 year olds were on-grade for their age (compared to 40 percent in the national cohort), 39.7 percent of those age 15 (19 percent comparatively), and 31.8 percent of the age 17 group (10 percent comparatively). For both groups repetition was most likely to occur at the end of SSA and again at Std 6 and 7. (9184:3).

An important variable identified in the study was socio-economic status (SES). Even within the ELC group, although they all came from the same neighborhood, there were SES differences, and this had an impact on children's school achievement. Those who attended the ELC could be divided into 3 groups (high, medium and low SES), with those in the high group coming from working class homes, with about one third of them below the poverty line when the children were at the ELC. Many of these were upwardly mobile and during the course of the study they moved out of Kewtown. The low group tended to include more families under stress. These sub-groups differed significantly in their school performance, despite the fact that they all attended the same pre-school programme. Those in the high and middle SES group scored significantly higher than national norms. And while those children in the lowest SES group performed better than the national average in terms of their scholastic progress, the differences were not significant.

In summarizing the entire study, the researchers note:

> Overall, taking all available evidence into consideration, we feel that it is justifiable to conclude that participation in the ELC programme did have a lasting effect on the scho-lastic achievement of these disadvantaged children...We think that their results show considerably better progress throughout their school careers than could be expected for children of their socioeconomic background. Much more research is needed to confirm these findings, but we would hypothesize, on the basis of our own results and the American longitudinal studies, that the lasting effects of preschool education programs are most apparent in high school, and also that effects vary according to socio-economic background. (1984:59)

One of the criticisms of the studies that have come from the USA and the UK is that the quality of the pre-
school experience for young children is at such a high standard in these settings, that the transferability of research results to other countries is highly questionable. It is important to note that while the ELC program had a definite curriculum, the ELC teachers had much lower qualifications (Standard 8 + 2 years) and at least twice as many children to work with in the classrooms (a ratio of 1:14) as their North American counterparts. Thus it can be concluded that it is possible to obtain a positive impact from less costly models of pre-school provision.

Source: Center for Education Policy Development and World Bank 1994.

Addressing the Intersecting Needs of Women and Children

In Sub-Saharan Africa, about 50 percent of women are working in wage-earning sectors. Actual labor force participation is certainly much higher if non-wage sectors are also included. Furthermore, the increasing survival of young children, the changes in family structure and child-rearing practices and urban-rural migration have increased the need and demand for new and better ways to care for and ensure the well-being of young children. Studies on women's labor force participation and child-care show that employed mothers are in greater need of, and more likely to send children to ECD programs (Lehrer 1983). Recent evidence from a Latin American country shows that when child-care is not available, mothers who wish to work will conceal the child's age and enroll under-age children in the first grade, exacerbating an already serious overcrowding problem for other children in this grade (Edwards, Gaston and Tunali 1995). Due to repetition and under-age and over-age school entries, for every 100 children expected in the first year of primary school in South Africa, actual enrollments are 150 for African children and 131 for colored. (National Education Policy Investigation: Early Childhood Educare Report 1992). The result is serious overcrowding for other children in this grade (Edwards and others 1995).

This is particularly relevant to Africa's vast expanding urban population, where many urban poor mothers cannot afford purchasing adequate child-care, and the absence of child-care prevents mothers from seeking more stable and higher-paying jobs. Provision of ECD services can increase women's productivity not only by freeing up their time to earn wages, but also by providing direct employment in child-care for qualified women. This is especially true for the adoption of home-based day care models.

Creating Synergistic Effects of Health, Nutrition, and Early Stimulation

Child development cannot be broken up into separate domains, nor reduced to the bureaucratic turf of one sectoral ministry or another. A child's learning capacity depends on an interactive process of health, nutrition, and child-care giver interaction. The latest research on the relationship between health, nutrition, and stimulation argues convincingly that an adequate food supply is not enough to ensure a child's development. Growth and development are fostered when all these variables are present within a caring environment. A 10-year study in Mexico has demonstrated the negative effect of severe malnutrition and lack of home stimulation on school readiness and language development (Chavez and Martinez 1981).

Early childhood development programs are a necessary *foundation* for the other programs such as primary schooling or health care to be effective. They should be seen neither as a 'trade-off' against, nor a mere complement to, other development programs. Combined programs take advantage of the interactive effects among health, nutrition, and early stimulation, with increased benefits at marginal cost. In addition, early childhood services can serve as vehicles for extending primary health care, food security, and other development programs.

A key challenge, though, is to find effective ways to *organize and finance* the task. The information about the cost per child of services is still lacking for developing countries, especially in Sub-Saharan Africa. Similarly, while there are various ways of financing early child development services, there is a lack of a systematic review on this topic. Given the limited existing resources in Sub-Saharan Africa, the means of financing ECD programs have to be either through making efficient use of the existing health, nutrition, and basic education programs, by mobilizing additional community resources, or by reallocating the current budget. In addition, one might consider subsidizing private provision through tax incentives and other innovative means and by promoting more private and voluntary (NGO sector) investments.

In the final analysis, early childhood development programs should be seen as the basic underpinning for Sub-Saharan Africa's future and the foundation of a healthy, prosperous, creative and competitive region. Children have the 'right' to be cherished, to be loved, well-fed, and stimulated. To care about Sub-Saharan Africa's future is to ensure that its children grow up in an environment where they can achieve this right.

ANNEX 1

A List Of Sub-Saharan African Countries

Angola
Benin
Botswana
Burkina Faso
Burundi
Cameroon
Cape Verde
Central African Republic
Chad
Comoros
Congo
Côte d'Ivoire
Djibouti
Equatorial Guinea
Ethiopia
Gabon

The Gambia
Ghana
Guinea
Guinea-Bissau
Kenya
Lesotho
Liberia
Madagascar
Malawi
Mali
Mauritania
Mauritius
Mozambique
Namibia
Niger
Nigeria

Rwanda
Sao Tome and Principe
Senegal
Seychelles
Sierra Leone
Somalia
South Africa
Sudan
Swaziland
Tanzania
Togo
Uganda
Zaire
Zambia
Zimbabwe

ANNEX 2

Key Social Sector Indicators for Child Welfare

	GNP per capita[a]	Infant Mortality[b]	School Enrollment (gross)[c]	Immuni-zation (DPT)[d]	Immuni-zation (Measles)[e]	Malnutrition (stunting)
	US$	per 1,000	%	%	%	%
ANGOLA[f]	970	124	31	30	47	
BENIN	420	110	31	75	67	
BOTSWANA	2,590	35	65	57	60	37[g]
BURKINA FASO	300	132	18	47	42	29[h]
BURUNDI	180	106	30	63	61	48[i]
CAMEROON	770	61	46	37	34	24[i]
CAPE VERDE	870	40	52	99	95	15[i]
CAR	390	105	35	60	69	
CHAD	200	122	27	13	19	13[j]
COMOROS	520	89	37	60	60	
CONGO	920	114	71	60	55	28[h]
CÔTE D'IVOIRE	630	91	37	50	52	17[i]
DJIBOUTI		115	19	41	42	22[i]
EQU. GUINEA	360	117		60	53	
ERITREA			20			
ETHIOPIA	100	122	13	28	22	64[i]
GABON	4,050	94	67	66	65	18[g]
GAMBIA, The	360	132	32	90	87	24[g]
GHANA	430	81	45	48	50	26[h]
GUINEA	510	133	21	70	70	
GUINEA-BISSAU	220	140	25	45	46	22[g]
KENYA	270	61	53	85	76	33[i]
LESOTHO	660	46	55	80	77	33[h]
LIBERIA[k]	490	142		20	38	37[g]
MADAGASCAR	240	93	31	64	52	51[h]
MALAWI	220	134	44	92	92	49[h]
MALI	300	130	14	46	51	24[i]
MAURITANIA	510	117	33	44	49	57[i]
MAURITIUS	2,980	18	58	97	94	22[i]
MOZAMBIQUE	80	162	23	49	62	
NAMIBIA	1,660	57	75	73	71	28[h]
NIGER	270	123	13	20	20	32[i]
NIGERIA	310	84	48	29	34	43[i]
RWANDA	200	117	38	85	81	48[h]

	GNP per capita[a]	Infant Mortality[b]	School Enrollment (gross)[c]	Immuni-zation (DPT)[d]	Immuni-zation (Measles)[e]	Malnutrition (stunting)
	US$	per 1,000	%	%	%	%
SAO TOME AND PRINCIPE	330	65		60	57	26[i]
SENEGAL	730	68	30	52	46	22[h]
SEYCHELLES	6,370	16		96	92	5[i]
SIERRA LEONE	140	143	31	63	67	35[h]
SOMALIA[f]	120	132	7	18	30	30[j]
SOUTH AFRICA	2,902	53	72	79	85	25[h]
SUDAN [l]	300	99	27	51	49	32[j]
SWAZILAND	1,050	108	66	89	85	30[h]
TANZANIA [l]	110	92	33	82	79	43[i]
TOGO	330	85	51	53	48	30[i]
UGANDA	190	122	35	73	73	45[i]
ZAIRE [m]	240	91	36	29	33	27
ZAMBIA	370	107	42	64	62	40[h]
ZIMBABWE	540	47	66	72	77	21[h]

a. *African Development Indicators* (1995), 1993 figures (except where indicated) using Atlas

b. *African Development Indicators* (1995), 1992 figures.

c. A Statistical Profile of Education in Sub-Saharan Africa 1990-93 UNESCO, enrollment ratio figures from 1990-93 (depending on country), based on 6-23 age group.

d. *African Development Indicators* (1995), 1993 figures based on 0-1 age group.

e. *African Development Indicators* (1995), 1993 figures based on 0-1 age group.

f. GNP is 1990 figure.

g. *Better Health for Africa* (1994), age group 24-59 mos. 1980-90.

h. WHO Global Database, various years

i. "The worldwide magnitude of protein-energy malnutrition: an overview from the WHO Global Database on Child Growth",- Bulletin of the World Health Organization, Vol. 71, number 6,-1993: pp. 703-712, various years.

j. *African Development Indicators* (1995).

k. GNP is 1987 figure.

l. GNP is 1992 figure

m. GNP is 1989 figure.

BIBLIOGRAPHY

African National Congress. 1994. *A Policy Framework for Education and Training.* South Africa.

Ainsworth, Martha, Mead Over, and A. A. Rwegarulira. 1992. *Economic Impact of AIDS on Orphaned Children: What Does the Evidence Show?* Washington, D.C.: World Bank. Prepared for the Expert Meeting on Family and Development, National Academy of Sciences, July 16-17, 1992 Washington, D.C.

Asomaning, V., S. Agarwal, N. Apt, M. Grieco and J. Turner. 1994. "The Missing Gender: An Explanation of the Low Enrollment Rates of Girls in Ghanaian Primary Schools." Mimeo. Washington D.C.: The World Bank.

Bernard Van Leer Foundation. 1985. *Reaching Children Where They Are.* Newsletter No. 80, October.

————. 1994. *Building on People's Strengths: Early Childhood in Africa.* The Hague.

Biersteker, Linda. 1994. "Early Childhood Educare Services for Black Children in South Africa." Report commissioned by the National Educare Forum, South Africa.

Center for Education Policy Development and World Bank. 1994. "Report of the South African Study on Early Childhood Development, Recommendations for Action in Support of Young Children." Johannesburg. August.

Chavez, A., and C. Martinez. 1981. "School Performance of Supplemented and Unsupplemented Children from a Poor Rural Area." In A. E. Harper and G. K. Davis (eds.), *Nutrition in Health and Disease and International Development: Symposia from the XII International Congress on Nutrition;* Vol. 77. New York: Alan R. Liss.

Colclough, C. 1980. 'Primary Schooling and Economic Development: A Review of the Evidence,' Washington D.C. Staff Working Paper No. 399. Washington, D.C.: World Bank.

Darlington, R. B., J. M. Royce, A. S. Snipper, H. W. Murray, and I. Lazar. 1980. 'Preschool programs and the later school competence of children from low-income families.' *Science* 208:202-204.

Edwards, J., N. Gaston, I. Tunali. 1995. *Under-age School Enrollment As Hidden Demand for Day Care.* Mimeo. Tulane University.

Evans, J. L. 1994. "Child Rearing Practices and beliefs in Sub-Saharan Africa." Report of a Workshop held in Windhoek, Namibia.

Fuller, B., P. Pillay, and N. Sirur. 1995. *Literacy Trends in South Africa: Expanding Education While Reinforcing Unequal Achievement?* Cape Town: University of Cape Town, Department of Economics.

Garcia, M. 1994. *Malnutrition and Food Insecurity Projections, 2020.* Washington, D.C.: International Food Policy Research Institute (IFPRI).

Glewwe, P., and Hanan Jacoby. 1992. Living Standards Measurement Study Working Paper No. 98. "Delayed Primary School Enrollment and Childhood Malnutrition in Ghana." Washington, D.C.: World Bank.

Grawe, R. 1979. 'Ability in Preschoolers, Earnings, and Home Environment.' Staff Working Paper No. 319. Washington, D.C.: World Bank.

Hubbell McKey, Ruth and others. 1985. *The Impact of Head Start on Children, Families, and Communities.* Washington, DC.: CSR Incorporated.

Hayes, Cheryl, John Palmer and Martha Zaslow. 1991. *Who Cares for America's Children?* Washington, D.C.: National Academy Press.

Lehrer, E. 1983. 'Determinants of Child Care Mode Choice: An Economic Perspective.' *Social Science Research* 12:69-80.

Levine, R. A., S. Dixon, S. Levine, A. Richman, P. H. Leiderman, C. H. Keefer, and T. B. Brazelton. 1994. *Child Care and Culture: Lessons from Africa.* Massachusetts: Cambridge University Press.

Levinger, B. 1994. *Nutrition, Health, and Education for All.* New York: UNDP.

———. 1995. *Critical Transitions: Human Capacity Development Across the Lifespan.* UNDP, New York.

Lockheed, M. E., D. Jamison, and L. Lau. 1980. 'Farmer Education and Farm Efficiency: A Survey.' *Economic Development and Cultural Change* 29: 37-76.

Lockheed, M. E. and Adriaan M. Verspoor. 1990. *Improving Primary Education in Developing Countries: A Review of Policy Options.* Washington, D.C.: World Bank.

Myers, R. G. 1992a. *The Twelve Who Survive.* London and New York: Routledge in cooperation with UNESCO.

———. 1992b. *Early Childhood Development Programs in Latin America: Toward Definition of an Investment Strategy.* Report No. 32, Human Resources Division, Latin America and the Caribbean Region, Washington D.C.: World Bank.

Norton, Andrew and Tom Stephens. 1995. *Participation in Poverty Assessments.* Participation Series. Environment Department. Washington, D.C.: World Bank.

Odaga, Adhiambo and Ward Heneveld. 1995. *Girls and Schooling in Sub-Saharan Africa.* World Bank Technical Paper No.296. Human Resources and Poverty Division, Africa Technical Department. Washington, D.C.: World Bank.

Olmsted, P., and D. Weikart. 1989. *How Nations Serve Young Children: Profiles of Child Care and Education in 14 Countries.* Michigan: The High/Scope Press.

Organization of African Unity and the United Nations Children's Fund. 1992a. *Africa's Children, Africa's Future: Human Investment Priorities for the 1990s.* Dakar, Senegal: OAU International Conference on Assistance to African Children.

———. 1992b. "Background Sectoral Papers." Dakar, Senegal: OAU International Conference on Assistance to African Children.

Psacharopoulos, G. and A.M. Arriagada. 1989. "Determinants of Early Age Human Capital Formation: Evidence from Brazil." *Economic Development and Cultural Change* 37: 683–708.

Psacharopoulos, G. 1995. *Building Human Capital for Better Lives.* Washington, D.C.: World Bank.

Rogoff, B. 1980. 'Schooling and the Development of Cognitive Skills,' In H. Triandis and A. Heron (eds.), *Handbook of Cross-cultural Psychology*, Vol. 4. Boston: Allyn-Bacon.

Schweinhart, L. J. and others. 1993. *Significant Benefits: The High/Scope Perry Preschool Study through Age 27.* Michigan: High/Scope Press.

Shaeffer, Sheldon. 1993. "The Impact of HIV/AIDS on Education Systems." *Educational Horizons* 71(4): 171-74.

Swaedner, Beth. 1994. "Kenya Early Childhood Development: Client Consultation Study." Eastern Africa Department: Washington, D.C.: World Bank.

Triandis, H. 1980. 'Reflections on Trends in Cross-cultural Research.' *Journal of Cross-cultural Psychology* 11: 35-58.

UNDP. 1994. *Human Development Report. 1994.* New York and Oxford: Oxford University Press and UNDP.

UNESCO. 1993. *Education for All: Status and Trends.* Paris.

———. 1992. Statistical Year Book, 1980-92. Paris.

UNHCR. 1993. *The State of the World's Refugees: The Challenge of Protection.* New York and London: Penguin Books.

UNICEF. 1991. *Challenges for Children and Women in the 1990s.* New York.

———. 1993. *Children and Women in South Africa.* New York.

———. 1994. *Situation Analysis of Women and Children in Mauritius 1994.* New York.

———. 1995. *The State of the World's Children.* New York.

Urasa, I. 1990. *Women and Rural Transport: An Assessment of Their Role in Sub-Saharan Africa.* Rural Travel and Transport Project, Sub-Sahara Africa Transport Program (SSATP), Technical Department, Africa Region. Washington, D.C.: World Bank.

U.S. Committee for Refugees. 1990. *World Refugee Survey 1990.* Washington, D.C.

Woodhead, Martin. 1995. "In Search of the Rainbow: Pathways to Quality in Large-Scale Programmes for Young Disadvantaged Children." Van Leer Foundation. Draft Mimeo. The Hague.

World Bank. 1992a. *Refugee and Displaced Women and Children in Sub-Saharan Africa.* AFTHR, *Information Sheet,* No. 2. Poverty and Human Resource Division, Technical Department, Africa Region. Washington, D.C.

———. 1992b. *Poverty in Sub-Saharan Africa: Progress Report on the Implementation of Assistance Strategies to Reduce Poverty.* Poverty and Human Resources Division, Technical Department, Africa Region. Washington, D.C.

———. 1993. *World Development Report 1993.* New York and Washington, D.C.: Oxford University Press and the World Bank.

———. 1994a. *World Development Report 1994.* New York and Washington, D.C.: Oxford University Press and the World Bank.

———. 1994b. "Human Resources Development in Africa: To Get Results on the Ground, Bank Strategies and Action." World Bank Internal Document. Poverty and Human Resources Division, Technical Department, Africa Region.

——— and the Government of Kenya. 1994c. *Kenya Welfare Monitoring Survey.* Eastern Africa Department. Washington, D.C.

———. 1994e. *Better Health in Africa: Experience and Lessons Learned.* Development in Practice Series. Washington, D.C.

———. 1995a. *African Development Indicators, (1994-95)* Private Sector Development and Economics Division, Technical Department Africa Region. Washington, D.C.

———. 1995b. *A Continent in Transition: Sub-Saharan African in the Mid-1990s.* Africa Region. Washington, D.C.

———. 1996. *Poverty in Sub-Saharan Africa.* Africa Technical Department. Washington, D.C.

Young, Mary E. 1995. Investing in Young Children. Discussion Paper No. 275. Washington, D.C.

————. 1996. Early Child Development, Investing in the Future. Directions in Development. Washington, D.C.

Distributors of World Bank Publications

Prices and credit terms vary from country to country. Consult your local distributor before placing an order.

ALBANIA
Adhion Ltd.
Perlat Rexhepi Str.
Pall. 9, Shk. 1, Ap. 4
Tirana
Tel: (42) 274 19; 221 72
Fax: (42) 274 19

ARGENTINA
Oficina del Libro Internacional
Av. Cordoba 1877
1120 Buenos Aires
Tel: (1) 815-8156
Fax: (1) 815-8354

AUSTRALIA, FIJI, PAPUA NEW GUINEA, SOLOMON ISLANDS, VANUATU, AND WESTERN SAMOA
D.A. Information Services
648 Whitehorse Road
Mitcham 3132
Victoria
Tel: (61) 3 9210 7777
Fax: (61) 3 9210 7788
URL: http://www.dadirect.com.au

AUSTRIA
Gerold and Co.
Graben 31
A-1011 Wien
Tel: (1) 533-50-14-0
Fax: (1) 512-47-31-29

BANGLADESH
Micro Industries Development Assistance Society (MIDAS)
House 5, Road 16
Dhanmondi R/Area
Dhaka 1209
Tel: (2) 326427
Fax: (2) 811188

BELGIUM
Jean De Lannoy
Av. du Roi 202
1060 Brussels
Tel: (2) 538-5169
Fax: (2) 538-0841

BRAZIL
Publicações Tecnicas Internacionais Ltda.
Rua Peixoto Gomide, 209
01409 Sao Paulo, SP.
Tel: (11) 259-6644
Fax: (11) 258-6990

CANADA
Renouf Publishing Co. Ltd.
1294 Algoma Road
Ottawa, Ontario K1B 3W8
Tel: 613-741-4333
Fax: 613-741-5439

CHINA
China Financial & Economic Publishing House
8, Da Fo Si Dong Jie
Beijing
Tel: (1) 333-8257
Fax: (1) 401-7365

COLOMBIA
Infoenlace Ltda.
Apartado Aereo 34270
Bogotá D.E.
Tel: (1) 285-2798
Fax: (1) 285-2798

COTE D'IVOIRE
Centre d'Edition et de Diffusion Africaines (CEDA)
04 B.P. 541
Abidjan 04 Plateau
Tel: 225-24-6510
Fax: 225-25-0567

CYPRUS
Center of Applied Research
Cyprus College
6, Diogenes Street, Engomi
P.O. Box 2006
Nicosia
Tel: 244-1730
Fax: 246-2051

CZECH REPUBLIC
National Information Center
prodejna, Konviktska 5
CS – 113 57 Prague 1
Tel: (2) 2422-9433
Fax: (2) 2422-1484
URL: http://www.nis.cz/

DENMARK
SamfundsLitteratur
Rosenoerns Allé 11
DK-1970 Frederiksberg C
Tel: (31)-351942
Fax: (31)-357822

EGYPT, ARAB REPUBLIC OF
Al Ahram
Al Galaa Street
Cairo
Tel: (2) 578-6083
Fax: (2) 578-6833

The Middle East Observer
41, Sherif Street
Cairo
Tel: (2) 393-9732
Fax: (2) 393-9732

FINLAND
Akateeminen Kirjakauppa
P.O. Box 23
FIN-00371 Helsinki
Tel: (0) 12141
Fax: (0) 121-4441
URL: http://booknet.cultnet.fi/aka/

FRANCE
World Bank Publications
66, avenue d'Iéna
75116 Paris
Tel: (1) 40-69-30-56/57
Fax: (1) 40-69-30-68

GERMANY
UNO-Verlag
Poppelsdorfer Allee 55
53115 Bonn
Tel: (228) 212940
Fax: (228) 217492

GREECE
Papasotiriou S.A.
35, Stournara Str.
106 82 Athens
Tel: (1) 364-1826
Fax: (1) 364-8254

HONG KONG, MACAO
Asia 2000 Ltd.
Sales & Circulation Department
Seabird House, unit 1101-02
22-28 Wyndham Street, Central
Hong Kong
Tel: 852 2530-1409
Fax: 852 2526-1107
URL: http://www.sales@asia2000.com.hk

HUNGARY
Foundation for Market Economy
Dombovari Ut 17-19
H-1117 Budapest
Tel: 36 1 204 2951 or 36 1 204 2948
Fax: 36 1 204 2953

INDIA
Allied Publishers Ltd.
751 Mount Road
Madras - 600 002
Tel: (44) 852-3938
Fax: (44) 852-0649

INDONESIA
Pt. Indira Limited
Jalan Borobudur 20
P.O. Box 181
Jakarta 10320
Tel: (21) 390-4290
Fax: (21) 421-4289

IRAN
Kowkab Publishers
P.O. Box 19575-511
Tehran
Tel: (21) 258-3723
Fax: 98 (21) 258-3723

Ketab Sara Co. Publishers
Khaled Eslamboli Ave.,
6th Street
Kusheh Delafrooz No. 8
Tehran
Tel: 8717819 or 8716104
Fax: 8862479
E-mail: ketab-sara@neda.net.ir

IRELAND
Government Supplies Agency
Oifig an tSoláthair
4-5 Harcourt Road
Dublin 2
Tel: (1) 461-3111
Fax: (1) 475-2670

ISRAEL
Yozmot Literature Ltd.
P.O. Box 56055
Tel Aviv 61560
Tel: (3) 5285-397
Fax: (3) 5285-397

R.O.Y. International
PO Box 13056
Tel Aviv 61130
Tel: (3) 5461423
Fax: (3) 5461442

Palestinian Authority/Middle East
Index Information Services
P.O.B. 19502 Jerusalem

ITALY
Licosa Commissionaria Sansoni SPA
Via Duca Di Calabria, 1/1
Casella Postale 552
50125 Firenze
Tel: (55) 645-415
Fax: (55) 641-257

JAMAICA
Ian Randle Publishers Ltd.
206 Old Hope Road
Kingston 6
Tel: 809-927-2085
Fax: 809-977-0243

JAPAN
Eastern Book Service
Hongo 3-Chome,
Bunkyo-ku 113
Tokyo
Tel: (03) 3818-0861
Fax: (03) 3818-0864
URL: http://www.bekkoame.or.jp/~svt-ebs

KENYA
Africa Book Service (E.A.) Ltd.
Quaran House, Mfangano Street
P.O. Box 45245
Nairobi
Tel: (2) 23641
Fax: (2) 330272

KOREA, REPUBLIC OF
Daejon Trading Co. Ltd.
P.O. Box 34
Yeoeida
Seoul
Tel: (2) 785-1631/4
Fax: (2) 784-0315

MALAYSIA
University of Malaya Cooperative Bookshop, Limited
P.O. Box 1127
Jalan Pantai Baru
59700 Kuala Lumpur
Tel: (3) 756-5000
Fax: (3) 755-4424

MEXICO
INFOTEC
Apartado Postal 22-860
14060 Tlalpan,
Mexico D.F.
Tel: (5) 606-0011
Fax: (5) 624-2822

NETHERLANDS
De Lindeboom/InOr-Publikaties
P.O. Box 202
7480 AE Haaksbergen
Tel: (53) 574-0004
Fax: (53) 572-9296

NEW ZEALAND
EBSCO NZ Ltd.
Private Mail Bag 99914
New Market
Auckland
Tel: (9) 524-8119
Fax: (9) 524-8067

NIGERIA
University Press Limited
Three Crowns Building Jericho
Private Mail Bag 5095
Ibadan
Tel: (22) 41-1356
Fax: (22) 41-2056

NORWAY
Narvesen Information Center
Book Department
P.O. Box 6125 Etterstad
N-0602 Oslo 6
Tel: (22) 57-3300
Fax: (22) 68-1901

PAKISTAN
Mirza Book Agency
65, Shahrah-e-Quaid-e-Azam
P.O. Box No. 729
Lahore 54000
Tel: (42) 7353601
Fax: (42) 7585283

Oxford University Press
5 Bangalore Town
Sharae Faisal
PO Box 13033
Karachi-75350
Tel: (21) 446307
Fax: (21) 454-7640
E-mail: oup@oup.khi.erum.com.pk

PERU
Editorial Desarrollo SA
Apartado 3824
Lima 1
Tel: (14) 285380
Fax: (14) 286628

PHILIPPINES
International Booksource Center Inc.
Suite 720, Cityland 10
Condominium Tower 2
H.V.dela Costa, corner
Valero St.
Makati, Metro Manila
Tel: (2) 817-9676
Fax: (2) 817-1741

POLAND
International Publishing Service
Ul. Piekna 31/37
00-577 Warzawa
Tel: (2) 628-6089
Fax: (2) 621-7255

PORTUGAL
Livraria Portugal
Rua Do Carmo 70-74
1200 Lisbon
Tel: (1) 347-4982
Fax: (1) 347-0264

ROMANIA
Compani De Librarii Bucuresti S.A.
Str. Lipscani no. 26, sector 3
Bucharest
Tel: (1) 613 9645
Fax: (1) 312 4000

RUSSIAN FEDERATION
Isdatelstvo <Ves Mir>
9a, Kolpachniy Pereulok
Moscow 101831
Tel: (95) 917 87 49
Fax: (95) 917 92 59

SAUDI ARABIA, QATAR
Jarir Book Store
P.O. Box 3196
Riyadh 11471
Tel: (1) 477-3140
Fax: (1) 477-2940

SINGAPORE, TAIWAN, MYANMAR, BRUNEI
Asahgate Publishing Asia Pacific Pte. Ltd.
41 Kallang Pudding Road #04-03
Golden Wheel Building
Singapore 349316
Tel: (65) 741-5166
Fax: (65) 742-9356
e-mail: ashgate@asianconnect.com

SLOVAK REPUBLIC
Slovart G.T.G. Ltd.
Krupinska 4
PO Box 152
852 99 Bratislava 5
Tel: (7) 839472
Fax: (7) 839485

SOUTH AFRICA, BOTSWANA
For single titles:
Oxford University Press
Southern Africa
P.O. Box 1141
Cape Town 8000
Tel: (21) 45-7266
Fax: (21) 45-7265

For subscription orders:
International Subscription Service
P.O. Box 41095
Craighall
Johannesburg 2024
Tel: (11) 880-1448
Fax: (11) 880-6248

SPAIN
Mundi-Prensa Libros, S.A.
Castello 37
28001 Madrid
Tel: (1) 431-3399
Fax: (1) 575-3998
http://www.tsai.es/mprensa

Mundi-Prensa Barcelona
Consell de Cent, 391
08009 Barcelona
Tel: (3) 488-3009
Fax: (3) 487-7659

SRI LANKA, THE MALDIVES
Lake House Bookshop
P.O. Box 244
100, Sir Chittampalam A. Gardiner Mawatha
Colombo 2
Tel: (1) 32105
Fax: (1) 432104

SWEDEN
Fritzes Customer Service
Regeringsgaton 12
S-106 47 Stockholm
Tel: (8) 690 90 90
Fax: (8) 21 4777

Wennergren-Williams AB
P. O. Box 1305
S-171 25 Solna
Tel: (8) 705-97-50
Fax: (8) 27-00-71

SWITZERLAND
Librairie Payot
Service Institutionnel
Côtes-de-Montbenon 30
1002 Lausanne
Tel: (021)-341-3229
Fax: (021)-341-3235

Van Diermen Editions Techniq
Ch. de Lacuez 41
CH1807 Blonay
Tel: (021) 943 2673
Fax: (021) 943 3605

TANZANIA
Oxford University Press
Maktaba Street
PO Box 5299
Dar es Salaam
Tel: (51) 29209
Fax: (51) 46822

THAILAND
Central Books Distribution
306 Silom Road
Bangkok
Tel: (2) 235-5400
Fax: (2) 237-8321

TRINIDAD & TOBAGO, JAM.
Systematics Studies Unit
#9 Watts Street
Curepe
Trinidad, West Indies
Tel: 809-662-5654
Fax: 809-662-5654

UGANDA
Gustro Ltd.
Medhvani Building
PO Box 9997
Plot 16/4 Jinja Rd.
Kampala
Tel/Fax: (41) 254763

UNITED KINGDOM
Microinfo Ltd.
P.O. Box 3
Alton, Hampshire GU34 2PG
England
Tel: (1420) 86848
Fax: (1420) 89889

ZAMBIA
University Bookshop
Great East Road Campus
P.O. Box 32379
Lusaka
Tel: (1) 213221 Ext. 482

ZIMBABWE
Longman Zimbabwe (Pte.)Ltd.
Tourle Road, Ardbennie
P.O. Box ST125
Southerton
Harare
Tel: (4) 6216617
Fax: (4) 621670